The Ultimate Wellness Book

The Ultimate Wellness Book

◆

Great tips for a healthier lifestyle

Sherman A. Moss

iUniverse, Inc.
New York Lincoln Shanghai

The Ultimate Wellness Book
Great tips for a healthier lifestyle

iUniverse books may be ordered through booksellers or by contacting:

iUniverse
2021 Pine Lake Road, Suite 100
Lincoln, NE 68512
www.iuniverse.com
1-800-Authors (1-800-288-4677)

ISBN-13: 978-0-595-39685-6 (pbk)
ISBN-13: 978-0-595-84091-5 (ebk)
ISBN-10: 0-595-39685-2 (pbk)
ISBN-10: 0-595-84091-4 (ebk)

Printed in the United States of America

Contents

Introduction

If you're like most Americans, you plan for your future. When you take a job, you examine its benefit plan. When you buy a home, you consider its location and condition so that your investment is safe. Today, more and more Americans are protecting their most important asset—their health. Are you?

Taking time out for exercise, using the food label to pick nutritious foods, taking advantage of the several fitness programs available, and getting needed medical attention can go a long way toward helping most people avoid the health pitfalls and fully enjoy their lives.

This book is a challenge to everyone who seeks to improve their health. The Ultimate Wellness Book prescription is a call to all health experts and professionals to continue to inform people that by learning about health and fitness, they will be empowered to rebuild and maintain their good health. Only by committing oneself to a healthier lifestyle will people change their ways. The Ultimate Wellness Book is a critical and necessary tool for everyone to learn, and believe in changing their health for the best.

Helping your overweight child

In the United States at least one child in five is overweight and the number of overweight children continues to grow. Over the last 2 decades, this number has increased by more than 50 percent, and the number of "extremely" overweight children has nearly doubled. A doctor determines if children are overweight by measuring their height and weight. Although children have fewer weight-related health problems than adults, overweight children are at high risk of becoming overweight adolescents and adults. Overweight adults are at risk for a number of health problems including heart disease, diabetes, high blood pressure stroke, and some forms of cancer.

Children become overweight for a variety of reasons. The most common causes are genetic factors, lack of physical activity, unhealthy eating patterns, or a combination of these factors. In rare cases, a medical problem, such as an endocrine disorder, may cause a child to become overweight. Your physician can perform a careful physical exam and some blood tests, if necessary, to rule out this type of problem.

Children whose parents or brothers or sisters are overweight may be at an increased risk of becoming overweight themselves. Although weight problems run in families, not all children with a family history of obesity will be overweight. Genetic factors play a role in increasing the likelihood that a child will be overweight, but shared family behaviors such as eating and activity habits also influence body weight.

A child's total diet and his or her activity level both play an important role in determining a child's weight. The increasing popularity of television and computer and video games contributes to children's inactive lifestyles. The average American child spends approximately 24 hours each week watching television-time that could be spent in some sort of physical activity.

If you think that your child is overweight, it is important to talk with your child's doctor. A doctor is the best person to determine whether your child has a weight problem. Physicians will measure your child's weight and height to determine if your child's weight is within a healthy range. A physician will also consider your child's age and growth patterns to determine whether your child is overweight. Assessing overweight in children is difficult because children grow in unpredictable spurts.

For example, it is normal for boys to have a growth spurt in weight and catch up in height later. It is best to let your child's doctor determine whether your child will "grow into" a normal weight. If your doctor finds that your child is overweight, he or she may ask you to make some changes in your family's eating and activity habits.

One of the most important things you can do to help overweight children is to let them know that they are okay whatever their weight. Children's feelings about themselves often are based on their parents' feelings about them. If you accept your children at any weight, they will be more likely to accept and feel good about themselves. It is also important to talk to your children about weight, allowing them to share their concerns with you. Your child probably knows better than anyone else that he or she has a weight problem. For this reason, overweight children need support, acceptance, and encouragement from their parents.

Parents should try not to set children apart because of their weight, but focus on gradually changing their family's physical activity and eating habits. Family involvement helps to teach everyone healthful habits and does not single out the overweight child.

Regular physical activity, combined with healthy eating habits, is the most efficient and healthful way to control your weight. It is also an important part of a healthy lifestyle. Some simple ways to increase your family's physical activity include the following:

Be a role model for your children. If your children see that you are physically active and have fun, they are more likely to be active and stay active for the rest of their lives.

Plan family activities that provide everyone with exercise and enjoyment, like walking, dancing, biking, or swimming. For example, schedule a walk with your family after dinner instead of watching TV.

Make sure that you plan activities that can be done in a safe environment.

Be sensitive to your child's needs. Overweight children may feel uncomfortable about participating in certain activity reduce the amount of time you and your family spend in sedentary activities, such as watching TV or playing video games. It is important to help your child find physical activities that they enjoy and that aren't embarrassing or too difficult.

The point is not to make physical activity an unwelcome chore, but to make the most of the opportunities you and your family have to be active.

Become more active throughout your day and encourage your family to do so as well. For example, walk up the stairs instead of taking the elevator, or do some activity during a work or school break-get up and stretch or walk around.

Teaching healthy eating practices early will help children approach eating with the right attitude-that food should be enjoyed and is necessary for growth, development, and for energy to keep the body running. The best way to begin is to learn more about children's nutritional needs by reading or talking with a health professional and then to offer them some healthy options, allowing your children to choose what and how much they eat.

Children should never be placed on a restrictive diet to lose weight, unless a doctor supervises one for medical reasons. Limiting what children eat may be harmful to their health and interfere with their growth and development.

Most of the foods in your diet should come from the grain products group (6-11 servings), the vegetable group (3-5 servings), and the fruit group (2-4 servings). Your diet should include moderate amounts of foods from the milk group (2-3 servings) and the meat and beans group (2-3 servings).

Foods that provide few nutrients and are high in fat and sugars should be used sparingly. Fat should not be restricted in the diets of children younger than 2 years of age.

If you are unsure about how to select and prepare a variety of foods for your family, consult a physician or registered dietitian for nutrition counseling.

Reducing fat is a good way to cut calories without depriving your child of nutrients. Simple ways to cut the fat in your family's diet include eating low fat or nonfat dairy products, poultry without skin and lean meats, and low fat or fat-free breads and cereals. Making small changes to the amount of fat in your family's diet is a good way to prevent excess weight gain in children: however, major efforts to change your child's diet should be supervised by a health professional. In addition, fat should not be restricted in the diets of children younger than 2 years of age. After that age, children should gradually adopt a diet that contains no more than 30 percent of calories from fat by the time the child is about 5 years old.

While it is important to be aware of the fat, salt, and sugar content of the foods you serve, all foods-even those that are high in fat or sugar-have a place in the diet, in moderation. Make a wide variety of healthful foods available in the house. This practice will help your children learn how to make healthy food choices.
Try to make mealtimes pleasant with conversation and sharing, not a time for scolding or arguing. If mealtimes are unpleasant, children may try to eat faster to leave the table as soon as possible. They then may learn to associate eating with stress.

These activities offer parents hints about children's food preferences, teach children about nutrition, and provide children with a feeling of accomplishment. In addition, children may be more willing to eat or try foods that they help prepare. Continuous snacking may lead to overeating, but snacks that are planned at specific times during the day can be part of a nutritious diet, without spoiling a child's appetite at mealtimes. You should make snacks as nutritious as possible, without depriving your child of occasional chips or cookies, especially at parties or other social events. Below are some ideas for healthy snacks.

Healthy Snacks

Fresh, frozen, or canned vegetables and fruit served either plain or with low fat or fat-free cheese or yogurt.
Dried fruit, served with nuts or sunflower or pumpkin seeds.
Breads and crackers made with enriched flour and whole grains, served with fruit spread or fat-free cheese.
Frozen desserts, such as nonfat or low fat ice cream, frozen yogurt, fruit sorbet, popsicles, water ice, and fruit juice bars.

Try to eat only in designated areas of your home, such as the dining room or kitchen. Eating in front of the TV may make it difficult to pay attention to feelings of fullness, and may lead to overeating.

Withholding food as a punishment may lead children to worry that they will not get enough food. For example, sending children to bed without any dinner may cause them to worry that they will go hungry. As a result, children may try to eat whenever they get a chance. Similarly, when foods, such as sweets, are used as a reward, children may assume that these foods are better or more valuable than other foods. For example, telling children that they will get dessert if they eat all of their vegetables sends the wrong message about vegetables.

Find out more about your school lunch program, or pack your child's lunch to include a variety of foods. Also, select healthier items when dining at restaurants.

Children are good learners, and they learn best by example. Setting a good example for your kids by eating a variety of foods and being physically active will teach your children healthy lifestyle habits that they can follow for the rest of their lives.

Look for the following characteristics when choosing a weight-control program for your child. The program should:

Be staffed with a variety of health professionals. The best programs may include exercise physiologists, pediatricians or family physicians, and psychiatrists or psychologists.

Perform a medical evaluation of the child. Before being enrolled in a program, your child's weight, growth, and health should be reviewed by a physician. During enrollment, your child's weight, growth, and health should be monitored by a health professional at regular intervals.

Focus on the whole family, not just the overweight child.

Be adapted to the specific age and capabilities of the child. Programs for 4-year-olds are different from those developed for children 8 or 12 years of age in terms of degree of responsibility of the child and parents.

Focus on behavioral changes.
Teach the child how to select a variety of foods in appropriate portions.

Encourage daily activity and limit sedentary activity, such as watching TV. Include a maintenance program and other support and referral resources to reinforce the new behaviors and to deal with underlying issues that contributed to overweight.

The overall goal of a successful treatment program should be to help the whole family focus on making healthy changes to their eating and activity habits that they will be able to maintain throughout life.

Fruits and Vegetables

"I know I should eat more fruits and vegetables. But how??"

"How can I get my kids to eat more vegetables?"

"Are oranges the only foods with vitamin C?"

Any of these questions sound familiar? Fruits and vegetables are key parts of your daily diet. Everyone needs 5 to 9 daily servings of fruits and vegetables for the nutrients they contain and for general health.

Nutrition and health may be reasons you eat certain fruits and vegetables, but there are many other reasons why you choose the ones you do. Perhaps it is because of taste, or physical characteristics such as crunchiness, juiciness, or bright colors.
You may eat some fruits and vegetables because of fond memories—like watermelon or corn at cookouts, your mom's green bean casserole, or tomatoes your dad brought in from the backyard garden. Or you may simply like them because most are quick to prepare and easy to eat.

Nutrition Tidbit

Fruits and vegetables give you many of the nutrients that you need: vitamins, minerals, dietary fiber, and water. Some are sources of let vitamin A, while others are rich in vitamin C, folate, or potassium. Almost all fruits and vegetables are naturally low in fat and calories and none have cholesterol. All of these healthful characteristics may protect you from getting chronic diseases, such as heart disease, stroke, and some types of cancer.

Fruits

Fruits taste great and they're bright and colorful, easy to find, and easy to prepare and eat. There are so many to choose from. Fruits are available in many different forms—fresh, frozen, canned, dried, and as juice. All are good ways to get the recommended 2 to 4 servings of fruits a day.

At breakfast, top your cereal with bananas or peaches; add blueberries to pancakes; drink 100% orange or grapefruit juice.

At lunch, pack a tangerine, banana, or grapes to eat, or choose fruits from a salad bar. Don't forget individual containers of fruits—they are easy and convenient. Kids think they're fun!

At dinner, add crushed pineapple to coleslaw; include mandarin oranges in a tossed salad; have a fruit salad for dessert.

For snacks, spread peanut butter on apple slices; have a frozen juice bar (100% juice); top frozen yogurt with berries or slices of kiwi fruit; snack on some dried fruit.

Vegetables

For some of us, summertime just wouldn't be the same without fresh produce. Maybe you garden or take trips to a local farmers market. Even your grocery store may have more fruits and vegetables in the summer. With vegetables, you and your family are getting delicious food and, nutritionally, you are getting many of the nutrients needed for good health vitamins, minerals, and dietary fiber.

Like fruits, vegetables are available not only fresh, but frozen, canned, dried, and as juice. You can eat them raw, steamed, boiled, stir-fried, grilled, micro waved, or baked. Aim for 3 to 5 servings of vegetables a day. Here are some ways you can jazz up vegetables to make them even more flavorful…to help you eat the servings you need.

Spice it!
Top corn or black beans with salsa or a dash of hot sauce.
Add garlic to mashed potatoes.
Add a dash of nutmeg to spinach dishes.

Slice it!
Add cooked, chopped onions to cooked peas.
Add sliced or diced vegetables to meatloaf, stews, or scrambled eggs.
Make a grated carrot salad.

Mix it!
Cook zucchini and stewed tomatoes together.
Mix green beans, Italian dressing, and almonds together.
Stir fry broccoli with chicken or beef.

Zap it!
Microwave broccoli and sprinkle on Parmesan cheese
Microwave a sweet potato with ground cloves or cinnamon on top.
Heat frozen mixed vegetables for a last-minute side dish.

Fruit and vegetable tips

Think about variety.
There are so many fruits and vegetables to choose from. Try berries, half a grapefruit, or dried apricots for dessert or snack. Add kidney beans or black-eyed peas to your next soup, stew, or salad.

Appeal to your senses.
Most people prefer crunchy foods over mushy ones. Enjoy raw fruits, and serve vegetables raw **Consider convenience.**

Nowadays, you can buy fruits and vegetables that are pre-cut and packaged for minimal preparation and quick eating. Pick up a bag of salad greens and some baby carrots and have a salad in seconds.
or lightly steamed. This will also help retain more of the valuable nutrients that may decrease during cooking.

Offer dips or dressings on the side.
Many fruits and vegetables taste great with a dip or dressing. Try low-fat yogurt or pudding as a dip for fruits like melons. Try low-fat salad dressing with raw broccoli, red and green peppers, or cauliflower.

Add vegetables to your favorite foods.
Shred carrots or zucchini into meatloaf or casseroles. Include chopped vegetables in pasta sauce or lasagna. Order a veggie pizza.

Keep fruits and vegetables around and "in sight."
Studies show that families that have fruits and vegetables around eat more of them. So, keep fruits and vegetables visible. Put a bowl of fruit on the table and keep cut-up carrot and celery sticks in a clear container in the refrigerator.

Think "salad."

Try a chef's salad for lunch, a fruit salad for dessert, or mixed greens along with your dinner. Many vegetables taste great in salads-try something different, like baby spinach, garbanzo beans, cauliflower, or red cabbage.

Use your blender.
Make a fruit smoothie by blending low-fat milk or yogurt with fresh or frozen fruit. Try strawberries, bananas, peaches, and other fruits.

Use fruits and vegetables as ingredients.
Try applesauce as a fat-free substitute for some of the oil when baking cakes. Add pureed, cooked vegetables to thicken stews and soups. These add additional flavors and textures to foods.

Snack on fruits and vegetables.
For a crunchy snack, try baby carrots or a crispy apple. For smooth and sweet, have a banana. Need a flavor jolt? Munch on dried apricots. Treat yourself to the luxury of fresh raspberries.

Helping kids enjoy more fruits and vegetables

It can be tough to get kids to eat a variety of fruits and vegetables. Don't force the foods, but continue to offer a variety. Try these ideas:

Set a good example by eating fruits and vegetables yourself. You are a role model for your kids in so many ways. Eating is no exception. When your kids see you eating and enjoying fruits and vegetables, they will too.

Offer lots of choices. Give children a choice of fruits for lunch. Let them help decide on the dinner vegetables. Kids enjoy helping in the kitchen, and are often more willing to eat foods they help choose and prepare. Depending on their ages, kids can help shop for, clean, and prepare fruits and vegetables into the salad.

Keep foods separate. Kids often prefer foods served separately. If they want to mix peas and corn, let them do it themselves.

Dietary fiber...for your health

We hear a lot about "dietary fiber" these days-and for good reason. Research suggests that it is important for proper bowel function by keeping us "regular." But what exactly is dietary fiber? It is the part of plants that the human digestive tract cannot break down. As a result, dietary fiber keeps waste moving through our intestines.

Most of us don't eat enough dietary fiber, and health experts suggest we eat more. Dry beans and peas are the best sources of fiber. There are a wide variety of these tasty foods in different sizes, shapes, flavors, and colors.

The Bottom Line

Remember "5 A Day": Aim for at least 2 servings of fruits and 3 servings of vegetables every day.

Build a good eating pattern, including fruits and vegetables, to ensure that you get all the nutrients you need for a healthy diet.

Choose whole or cut-up fruits and vegetables rather than juices most often; juices contain little or no dietary fiber.

Set good eating examples for your children.

Four Simple Steps to Food Safety

Right now, there may be an invisible enemy ready to strike. He's called bacteria and it can make you and those you care about sick. In fact, even though you can't see bacteria—or smell it, or feel it—it and millions more like it may have already invaded the food you eat.

But you have the power to fight bacteria and to keep you food safe from harmful bacteria. It's as easy as following these four simple steps:

Clean: Wash hand and surfaces often

Bacteria can spread throughout the kitchen and get onto cutting boards, utensils, sponges and counter tops. Here's how to fight bacteria:

- Wash your hands with hot soapy water before handling food and after using the bathroom, changing diapers and handling pets.

- Wash your cutting boards, dishes, utensils and counter topes with hot soapy water after preparing each food item and before you go on to the next food.

- Use plastic or other non-porous cutting boards. These boards should be run through the dishwasher—or washed in hot soapy water—after use

- Consider using paper towels to clean up kitchen surfaces. If you use cloth towels, wash them often in the hot cycle or your washing machine.

Separate: Don't cross-contaminate

Cross-contaminate is the scientific word for how bacteria can be spread from one food product to another. This is especially true when handling raw meat, poultry and seafood, so keep these foods and their juices away from ready-to-eat foods. Here's how to fight bacteria:

- Separate raw meat, poultry and seafood from other foods in your grocery shopping cart and in your refrigerator.

- If possible, use a different cutting board for raw meat products.

- Always wash hands, cutting boards, dishes and utensils with hot soapy water after they come in contact with raw meat, poultry and seafood.

- Never place cooked food on a plate which previously held raw meat, poultry and seafood.

Cook: Cook to proper temperatures

Food safety experts agree that foods are properly cooked when they are heated for a long enough time and at a high enough temperature to kill the harmful bacteria that cause food borne illness.
The best way to fight bacteria:

- Use a clean thermometer, which measures the internal temperature of cooked foods, to make sure meat, poultry, casseroles and other foods are cooked all the way through.

- Cook roasts and steaks to at least 145 F. Whole poultry should be cooked to 180 F for doneness.

- Cook eggs until the yolk and white are firm. Don't use recipes in which eggs remain raw or only partially cooked.

- Fish should be opaque and flake easily with a fork.

- When cooking in a microwave oven, make sure there are no cold spots in food where bacteria can survive. For best results, cover food, stir and rotate for even cooking. If there is no turntable, rotate the dish by hand once or twice during cooking.

- Bring sauces, soups and gravy to a boil when reheating. Heat other leftovers thoroughly to at least 165 F.

Chill: Refrigerate promptly

Refrigerate foods quickly because cold temperatures keep harmful bacteria from growing and multiplying. So, set your refrigerator no higher than 40 F and the freezer unit at 0 F. Check these temperatures occasionally with an appliance thermometer. Then, fight bacteria by following these steps:

- Refrigerate or freeze perishables, prepared foods and leftovers within two hours or sooner.

- Never defrost food at room temperature. Thaw food in the refrigerator, under cold running water or in the microwave. Marinate foods in the refrigerator.

- Divide large amounts of leftovers into small, shallow containers for quick cooling in the refrigerator.

- Don't pack the refrigerator. Cool air must circulate to keep food safe.

Although an invisible enemy may be in your kitchen, you have four powerful tools to fight bacteria: washing hands and surfaces often, avoiding cross-contamination, cooking to proper temperatures, and refrigerating promptly. So, be a bacteria fighter and make the meals and snacks from your kitchen as safe as possible.

How Much Are You Eating

"Make that mega-sized."

"I'll have the gigantic-gulp."

"I don't believe I ate the whole thing!"

Many people feel that the bigger the portion, the better. But is that so? Not if you're trying to manage your weight. One key to getting or keeping your weight in a healthy range is to eat sensible portions. That's easy to say-but not always so easy to do! This book gives tips to help you decide what sensible portions are for you, and to help you stick to those reasonable portion sizes.

How much do you eat?

Suppose you had dinner at an Italian restaurant last night. You ordered spaghetti with meatballs. While you were waiting for your order, you ate 2 slices of garlic bread. How can you tell if this dinner is too much food for you?

Think about your plateful of spaghetti and meatballs. Estimate the amounts of spaghetti, sauce, and meat. You may decide, for example, that the spaghetti portion was about 2 cups, the tomato sauce looked like about 1 cup, and the meatballs were about 6 ounces. With the 2 slices of garlic bread, you now have an idea about how much you ate for dinner. But how do your portions translate into standard servings?

The number of servings from each food group depends on your calorie needs.

Children ages 2 to 6 years, many inactive women, and some older adults may need about 1,600 calories per day.

Most children over 6, teen girls, active women, and many inactive men may need about 2,200 calories per day.

Teen boys and active men may need about 2,800 calories per day.

For example, if you need about 1,600 calories a day, the recommendation is 6 daily servings from the Grains (Bread, Cereal, Rice & Pasta) group. How does this compare to your spaghetti dinner? Your dinner had 6 servings the total daily recommendation for someone with your calorie needs. If you had counted your portions of spaghetti and bread as only 1 serving each, you might think you had only eaten 2 servings from the Grains group. But, you actually ate 6! By comparing the portion you ate with a standard serving, you can judge whether your daily intake is right for you.

Serving sizes and the recommended number of servings from each group are guides to help determine your daily intake. Your portions do not have to match the standard serving size-they can be larger or smaller. But, the amount you eat over the day should match the total amount of a food that is recommended. Often, the food portions of grains and meats that people choose are larger than the normal serving size. Be especially careful when counting servings from these groups to figure out how many servings are in your portions.

Portions and servings—What's the difference?

A **portion** is the amount of food you choose to eat. There is no standard portion size and no single right or wrong portion size.

A **serving** is a standard amount used to help give advice about how much to eat, or to identify how many calories and nutrients are in a food.

Tips to help you choose sensible portions

When eating out:

Choose a "small" or "medium" portion. This includes main dishes, side dishes, and beverages as well. Remember that water is always a good option for quenching your thirst.

If main dish portions are larger than you want, order an appetizer or side dish instead, or share a main dish with a friend.

Resign from the "clean your plate club"-when you've eaten enough, leave the rest. If you can chill the extra food right away, take it home in a "doggie bag." Ask for salad dressing to be served "on the side" so you can add only as much as you want.

Order an item from the menu instead of the "all-you-can-eat" buffet.

At home:

Once or twice, measure your typical portion of foods you eat often. Use standard measuring cups. This will help you estimate the portion size of these foods and similar foods.

Be especially careful to limit portions of foods high in calories, such as cookies, cakes, other sweets, and fats, oils, and spreads.

Try using a smaller plate for your meal.

Put sensible portions on your plate at the beginning of the meal, and don't take "seconds."

The Bottom Line

Choosing sensible portions is a key to controlling calorie intake and getting or keeping your weight in a healthy range. What is sensible for you?

Each day, choose the recommended amount from the five food groups-depending on your calorie needs.

A serving may not be the same as the portion you choose to eat-compare to find out how many servings are in your portion.

Keep sensible portions in mind at restaurants as well as at home.

Revealing Trans Fats

Scientific evidence shows that consumption of saturated fat, *trans* fat, and dietary cholesterol raises low-density lipoprotein (LDL), or "bad" cholesterol, levels, which increases the risk of coronary heart disease (CHD). According to the National Heart, Lung, and Blood Institute of the National Institutes of Health, more than 12.5 million Americans have CHD, and more than 500,000 die each year. That makes CHD one of the leading causes of death in the United States. The Food and Drug Administration has required that saturated fat and dietary cholesterol be listed on food labels. With *trans* fat added to the Nutrition Facts panel, you will know for the first time how much of all three—saturated fat, *trans* fat, and cholesterol—are in the foods you choose. Identifying saturated fat, *trans* fat, and cholesterol on the food label gives you information you need to make food choices that help reduce the risk of CHD. This revised label will be of particular interest to people concerned about high blood cholesterol and heart disease. However, everyone should be aware of the risk posed by consuming too much saturated fat, *trans* fat, and cholesterol. But what is *trans* fat, and how can you limit the amount of this fat in your diet?

What is *Trans* Fat?

Basically, *trans* fat is made when manufacturers add hydrogen to vegetable oil—a process called hydrogenation. Hydrogenation increases the shelf life and flavor stability of foods containing these *Trans* fat can be found in vegetable shortenings, some margarines, crackers, cookies, snack foods, and other foods made with or fried in partially hydrogenated oils. Unlike other fats, the majority of *trans* fat is formed when food manufacturers turn liquid oils into solid fats like shortening and hard margarine. A small amount of *trans* fat is found naturally, primarily in dairy products, some meat, and other animal-based foods.

Trans fat, like saturated fat and dietary cholesterol, raises the LDL cholesterol that increases your risk for CHD. Americans consume on average 4 to 5 times as much saturated fat as *trans* fat in their diets.

Although saturated fat is the main dietary culprit that raises LDL, *trans* fat and dietary cholesterol also contribute significantly.

Are All Fats the Same?

Simply put: No. Fat is a major source of energy for the body and aids in the absorption of vitamins A, D, E, and K, and carotenoids. Both animal- and plant-derived food products contain fat, and when eaten in moderation, fat is important for proper growth, development, and maintenance of good health. As a food ingredient, fat provides taste, consistency, and stability and helps you feel full. In addition, parents should be aware that fats are an especially important source of calories and nutrients for infants and toddlers (up to 2 years of age), who have the highest energy needs per unit of body weight of any age group.

While unsaturated fats (monounsaturated and polyunsaturated) are beneficial when consumed in moderation, saturated and *trans* fats are not. Saturated fat and *trans* fat raise LDL cholesterol levels in the blood. Dietary cholesterol also raises LDL cholesterol and may contribute to heart disease even without raising LDL. Therefore, it is advisable to choose foods low in saturated fat, *trans* fat, and cholesterol as part of a healthful diet.

What Can You Do About Saturated Fat, *Trans* Fat, and Cholesterol?

When comparing foods, look at the Nutrition Facts panel, and choose the food with the lower amounts of saturated fat, *trans* fat, and cholesterol. Health experts recommend that you keep your intake of saturated fat, *trans* fat, and cholesterol as low as possible while consuming a nutritionally adequate diet. However, these experts recognize that eliminating these three components entirely from your diet is not practical because they are unavoidable in ordinary diets.

Where Can You Find *Trans* Fat on the Food Label?

Although some food products already have *trans* fat on the label, food manufacturers have to list it on all their products.

You will find *trans* fat listed on the Nutrition Facts panel directly under the line for saturated fat.

Do Dietary Supplements Contain *Trans* Fat?

Would it surprise you to know that some dietary supplements contain *trans* fat from partially hydrogenated vegetable oil as well as saturated fat or cholesterol?

It's true. As a result of the FDA's new label requirement, if a dietary supplement contains a reportable amount of *trans* or saturated fat, which is 0.5 gram or more, dietary supplement manufacturers must list the amounts on the Supplement Facts panel. Some dietary supplements that may contain saturated fat, *trans* fat, and cholesterol include energy and nutrition bars.

Fat Tips

Here are some practical tips you can use every day to keep your consumption of saturated fat, *trans* fat, and cholesterol low while consuming a nutritionally adequate diet.

Choose foods lower in saturated fat, *trans* fat, and cholesterol. For saturated fat and cholesterol, keep in mind that 5 percent of the daily value (%DV) or less is low and 20 percent or more is high. (There is no %DV for *trans* fat.) Choose alternative fats. Replace saturated and *trans* fats in your diet with monounsaturated and polyunsaturated fats. These fats do not raise LDL cholesterol levels and have health benefits when eaten in moderation. Sources of monounsaturated fats include olive and canola oils. Sources of polyunsaturated fats include soybean oil, corn oil, sunflower oil and foods like nuts and fish.

Choose vegetable oils (except coconut and palm kernel oils) and soft margarines (liquid, tub, or spray) more often because the amounts of saturated fat, *trans* fat, and cholesterol are lower than the amounts in solid shortenings, hard margarines, and animal fats, including butter.
Consider fish. Most fish are lower in saturated fat than meat. Some fish, such as mackerel, sardines, and salmon, contain omega-3 fatty acids that are being studied to determine if they offer protection against heart disease.

Ask before you order when eating out. A good tip to remember is to ask which fats are being used in the preparation of your food when eating or ordering out.

Watch calories. Don't be fooled! Fats are high in calories. All sources of fat contain 9 calories per gram, making fat the most concentrated source of calories. By comparison, carbohydrates and protein have only 4 calories per gram.

To keep your intake of saturated fat, *trans* fat, and cholesterol low:

Look at the Nutrition Facts panel when comparing products. Choose foods low in the combined amount of saturated fat and *trans* fat and low in cholesterol as part of a nutritionally adequate diet.

Substitute alternative fats that are higher in mono- and polyunsaturated fats like olive oil, canola oil, soybean oil, corn oil, and sunflower oil.

Highlights of the Final Rule on *Trans* Fat

Manufacturers of conventional foods and some dietary supplements will be required to list *trans* fat on a separate line, immediately under saturated fat on the nutrition label.

Food manufacturers have to list *trans* fat on the nutrition label. The regulatory chemical definition for *trans* fatty acids is all unsaturated fatty acids that contain one or more isolated (i.e., non-conjugated) double bonds in a *trans* configuration. Dietary supplement manufacturers must also list *trans* fat on the Supplement Facts panel when their products contain reportable amounts (0.5 gram or more) of *trans* fat. Examples of dietary supplements with *trans* fat are energy and nutrition bars.

Facts about sugary snacks

Sugary snacks taste so good-but they aren't so good for your teeth or your body. The candies, cakes, cookies, and other sugary foods that kids love to eat between meals can cause tooth decay. Some sugary foods have a lot of fat in them too.

Kids who consume sugary snacks eat many different kinds of sugar every day, including table sugar (sucrose) and corn sweeteners (fructose). Starchy snacks can also break down into sugars once they're in your mouth.

Did you know that the average American eats about 147 pounds of sugars a year? That's a big pile of sugar! No wonder the average 17-year-old in this country has more than three decayed teeth!

Invisible germs called bacteria live in your mouth all the time. Some of these bacteria form a sticky material called plaque on the surface of the teeth. When you put sugar in your mouth, the bacteria in the plaque gobble up the sweet stuff and turn it into acids. These acids are powerful enough to dissolve the hard enamel that covers your teeth. That's how cavities get started. If you don't eat much sugar, the bacteria can't produce as much of the acid that eats away enamel.

Before you start munching on a snack, ask yourself what's in the food you've chosen. Is it loaded with sugar? If it is, think again. Another choice would be better for your teeth. And keep in mind that certain kinds of sweets can do more damage than others. Gooey or chewy sweets spend more time sticking to the surface of your teeth. Because sticky snacks stay in your mouth longer than foods that you quickly chew and swallow, they give your teeth a longer sugar bath.

You should also think about when and how often you eat snacks. Do you nibble on sugary snacks many times throughout the day, or do you usually just have dessert after dinner? Damaging acids form in your mouth every time you eat a sugary snack. The acids continue to affect your teeth for at least 20 minutes before they are neutralized and can't do any more harm. So, the more times you eat sugary snacks during the day, the more often you feed bacteria the fuel they need to cause tooth decay.

If you eat sweets, it's best to eat them as dessert after a main meal instead of several times a day between meals. Whenever you eat sweets—in any meal or snack—brush your teeth well with a fluoride toothpaste afterward.

When you're deciding about snacks, think about:

- the number of times a day you eat sugary snacks

- how long the sugary food stays in your mouth

- the texture of the sugary food (chewy? sticky?)

If you snack after school, before bedtime, or other times during the day, choose something without a lot of sugar or fat. There are lots of tasty, filling snacks that are less harmful to your teeth—and the rest of your body—than foods loaded with sugars and low in nutritional value.
Snack smart!

Low-fat choices like raw vegetables, fresh fruits, or whole-grain crackers or bread are smart choices. Eating the right foods can help protect you from tooth decay and other diseases. Next time you reach for a snack, pick a food from the list inside or make up your own menu of non-sugary, low-fat snack foods from the basic food groups.

Candy bars aren't the only culprits. Foods such as pizza, breads, and hamburger buns may also contain sugars. Check the label. The new food labels identify sugars and fats on the Nutrition Facts panel on the package. Keep in mind that brown sugar, honey, molasses, and syrups also react with bacteria to produce acids, just as refined table sugar does. These foods also are potentially damaging to teeth.

Your child's meals and snacks should include a variety of foods from the basic food groups, including fruits and vegetables; grains, including breads and cereals; milk and dairy products; and meat, nuts, and seeds. Some snack foods have greater nutritional value than others and will better promote your child's growth and development. However, be aware that even some fresh fruits, if eaten in excess, may promote tooth decay. Children should brush their teeth with fluoride toothpaste after snacks and meals. (So should you!)

Control Weight While Quitting Smoking

Not everyone gains weight when they stop smoking. On average, people who quit smoking gain only about 10 pounds. You are more likely to gain weight when you stop smoking if you have smoked for 10 to 20 years or smoked one or more packs of cigarettes a day. You can control your weight while you quit smoking by making healthy eating and physical activity a part of your life. Although you might gain a few pounds, remember you have stopped smoking and taken a big step toward a healthier life.

What causes weight gain after quitting?

When nicotine, a chemical in cigarette smoke, leaves your body, you may experience:
Short-term weight gain. The nicotine kept your body weight low, and when you quit smoking, your body returns to the weight it would have been had you never smoked.
You might gain 3 to 5 pounds due to water retention during the first week after quitting. A need for fewer calories. After you stop smoking, you may use fewer calories than when you were smoking.

Will this weight gain hurt my health?

The health risks of smoking are far greater than the risks of gaining 5 to 10 pounds. Smoking causes more than 400,000 deaths each year in the United States. You would have to gain about 100 to 150 pounds after quitting to make your health risks as high as when you smoked. The health risks of smoking and the benefits of quitting are listed below.

When you smoke...

Your heart rate increases. You are much more likely to get lung cancer than a nonsmoker. Men are 22 times more likely to develop lung cancer, while women who smoke are 12 times more likely.
You expose yourself to some 4,000 chemicals in cigarette smoke and 40 of these chemicals cause cancer.
You are twice as likely to have a heart attack as a nonsmoker.
You increase your risk for heart disease, stroke, some types of cancer, emphysema, chronic bronchitis, and other lung diseases.
You are hurting not only your own health, but the health of anyone who breathes the smoke, including nonsmokers.

When you quit smoking...

Your body begins to heal from the effects of the nicotine within 12 hours after your last cigarette.
Your heart and lungs start repairing the damage caused by cigarette smoke.
You breathe easier and your smoker's cough starts to go away.
You lower your risk for illness and death from heart disease, stroke, chronic bronchitis, emphysema, lung cancer, and other types of cancer.
You contribute to cleaner air, especially for children who are at risk for illnesses because they breathe others' cigarette smoke.

What Can I Do to Avoid Gaining Weight When I Quit Smoking?

To avoid gaining weight when you quit smoking, you need to become more physically active and improve your eating habits *before* you stop. Physical activity helps to control your weight by increasing the number of calories your body uses. Making healthy changes to your eating habits will prevent weight gain by controlling the amount of calories you eat. Try to reduce your chances of gaining weight by being more physically active and improving your eating habits *before* you stop smoking.

Become More Physically Active.

Becoming physically active is a healthy way to control your weight and take your mind off smoking. In one study, women who stopped smoking and added 45 minutes of walking a day gained less than 3 pounds. In addition to helping control your weight, exercise increases your energy, promotes self-confidence, improves your health, and may help relieve the stress and depression caused by the lack of nicotine in your body.

You can become more physically active by spending less time doing activities that use little energy, like watching television and playing video games, and spending more time doing physical activities. Try to do at least 30 minutes of physical activity a day on most days of the week. The activity does not have to be done all at once. It can be done in short spurts—10 minutes here, 20 minute there—as long as it adds up to 30 minutes a day. Simple ways to become more physically active include gardening, housework, mowing the lawn, playing actively with children, and taking the stairs instead of the elevator.

Improve Your Eating Habits.
Try to gradually improve your eating habits. Changing your eating habits too quickly can add to the stress you may feel as you try to quit smoking. Eating a variety of foods is a good way to improve your health. The Nutrition Facts Label that is found on most processed food products can also help you select foods that meet your daily nutritional needs.

Eat plenty of grain products, vegetables, and fruits.
Choose lean and low fat foods and low-calorie beverages most often. Choose low fat dairy products, lean meats, fish, poultry, and dry beans to get the nutrients you need without extra calories and fat.

Choose less often foods high in fat and sugars and low in nutrients.

When You Are Ready to Quit Smoking

Pick a day to quit smoking during a non-stressful period. For example, try not to quit smoking during holiday seasons when you might be tempted to eat more. Quitting during a stressful time at work or at home might cause extra snacking or a smoking relapse.
Try to focus on quitting smoking and healing your body. Your first goal should be to quit smoking and let your body heal from the effects of nicotine.

After you feel better and are not smoking, work harder on improving your eating and physical activity habits to help you lose any weight that you might have gained.

Weight Loss For Life

Who should lose weight? Health experts generally agree that adults can benefit from weight loss if they are moderately to severely overweight. Health experts also agree that adults who are overweight and have weight-related medical problems or a family history of such problems can benefit from weight loss. Some weight-related health problems include diabetes, heart disease, high blood pressure, high cholesterol levels, or high blood sugar levels. Even a small weight loss of 10 to 20 pounds can improve your health, for example by lowering your blood pressure and cholesterol levels. You do not need to lose weight if your weight is within the healthy range on the weight-for-height chart, you have gained less than 10 pounds since you reached your adult height, and you are otherwise healthy.

How We Lose Weight

Your body weight is controlled by the number of calories you eat and the number of calories you use each day. So, to lose weight you need to take in fewer calories than you use. You can do this by becoming more physically active or by eating less. Following a weight-loss program that helps you to become more physically active and decrease the amount of calories that you eat is most likely to lead to successful weight loss. The weight-loss program should also help you keep the weight off by making changes in your physical activity and eating habits that you will be able to follow for the rest of your life.

Types of Weight-Loss Programs

To lose weight and keep it off, you should be aware of the different types of programs available and the important parts of a good program. Knowing this information should help you select or design a weight-loss program that will work for you. The three types of weight-loss programs include: do-it-yourself programs, non-clinical programs, and clinical programs.

Do-It-Yourself Programs

Any effort to lose weight by yourself or with a group of like-minded others through support groups, worksite or community-based programs fits in the "do-it-yourself" category. Individuals using a do-it-yourself program rely on their own judgment, group support, and products such as diet books for advice.

Non-Clinical Programs

These programs may or may not be commercially operated, such as through a privately-owned, weight-loss chain. They often use books and pamphlets that are prepared by health-care providers. These programs use counselors (who usually are not health-care providers and may or may not have training) to provide services to you. Some programs require participants to use the program's food or supplements.

Clinical Programs

This type of program may or may not be commercially owned. Services are provided in a health-care setting, such as a hospital, by licensed health professionals, such as physicians, nurses, dietitians, and/or psychologists. In some clinical programs, a health professional works alone; in others, a group of health professionals works together to provide services to patients. Clinical programs may offer you services such as nutrition education, medical care, behavior change therapy, and physical activity.

Clinical programs may also use other weight-loss methods, such as very low-calorie diets, prescription weight-loss drugs, and surgery, to treat severely overweight patients. These treatments are described below:

Very low-calorie diets (VLCDs) are commercially prepared formulas that provide no more than 800 calories per day and replace all usual food intake. VLCDs help individuals lose weight more quickly than is usually possible with low-calorie diets.

Prescribed weight-loss drugs should be used only if you are likely to have health problems caused by your weight. You should not use drugs to improve your appearance. Prescribed weight-loss drugs, when combined with a healthy diet and regular physical activity, may help some obese adults lose weight. However, before these medications can be widely recommended, more research is needed to determine their long-term safety and effectiveness. Whatever the results, prescription weight-loss drugs should be used only as part of an overall program that includes long-term changes in your eating and physical activity habits.

You may consider gastric surgery to promote weight loss if you are more than 80 pounds overweight. The surgery, sometimes called bariatric surgery, causes weight loss in one of two ways:

1) by limiting the amount of food your stomach can hold by closing off or removing parts of the stomach or 2) by causing food to be poorly digested by bypassing the stomach or part of the intestines. After surgery, patients usually lose weight quickly. While some weight is often regained, many patients are successful in keeping off most of their weight. In some cases, the surgery can lead to problems that require follow-up operations. Surgery may also reduce the amount of vitamins and minerals in your body and cause gallstones.

If you are considering a weight-loss program and you have medical problems, or if you are severely overweight, programs run by trained health professionals may be best for you. These professionals are more likely to monitor you for possible side effects of weight loss and to talk to your doctor when necessary.
Whether you decide to use the do-it-yourself, non-clinical, or clinical approach, the program should help you lose weight and keep it off by teaching you healthy eating and physical activity habits that you will be able to follow for the rest of your life.

Diet

The word "diet" probably brings to mind meals of lettuce and cottage cheese. By definition, "diet" refers to what a person eats or drinks during the course of a day. A diet that limits portions to a very small size or that excludes certain foods entirely to promote weight loss may not be effective over the long term. Rather, you are likely to miss certain foods and find it difficult to follow this type of diet for a long time. Instead, it is often helpful to gradually change the types and amounts of food you eat and maintain these changes for the rest of your life. The ideal diet is one that takes into account your likes and dislikes and includes a wide variety of foods with enough calories and nutrients for good health.
How much you eat and what you eat play a major role in how much you weigh. So, when planning your diet, you should consider: What calorie level is appropriate? Is the diet you are considering nutritionally balanced? Will the diet be practi-

cal and easy to follow? Will you be able to maintain this eating plan for the rest of your life? The following information will help you answer these questions.

Calorie Level

Low-calorie Diets. Most weight-loss diets provide 1,000 to 1,500 calories per day. However, the number of calories that is right for you depends on your weight and activity level. At these calorie levels, diets are referred to as low-calorie diets. Self-help diet books and clinical and non-clinical weight-loss programs often include low-calorie diet plans.

The calorie level of your diet should allow for a weight loss of no more than 1 pound per week (after the first week or two when weight loss may be more rapid because of initial water loss). If you can estimate how many calories you eat in a day, you can design a diet plan that will help you lose no more than 1 pound per week. You may need to work with a trained health professional, such as a registered dietitian. Or, you can use a standardized low-calorie diet plan with a fixed calorie level.

The selected calorie level, however, may not produce the recommended rate of weight loss, and you may need to eat more or less.

Good Nutrition

Make sure that your diet contains all the essential nutrients for good health. Using the Nutrition Facts Label that is found on most processed food products can help you choose a healthful diet. The Nutrition Facts Label will help you select foods that meet your daily nutritional needs. A healthful diet should include:

Adequate vitamins and minerals. Eating a wide variety of foods from all the food groups will help you get the vitamins and minerals you need. If you eat less than 1,200 calories per day, you may benefit from taking a daily vitamin and mineral supplement.

Adequate protein. The average woman 25 years of age and older should get 50 grams of protein each day, and the average man 25 years of age and older should get 63 grams of protein each day. Adequate protein is important because it prevents muscle tissue from breaking down and repairs all body tissues such as skin and teeth. To get adequate protein in your diet, make sure you eat 2-3 servings from the Meat, Poultry, Fish, Dry Beans, Eggs, and Nuts Group. These foods are all good sources of protein.

Adequate carbohydrates. At least 100 grams of carbohydrates per day are needed to prevent fatigue and dangerous fluid imbalances. To make sure you get enough carbohydrates, eat 6-11 servings from the Bread, Cereal, Rice, and Pasta Group.

A daily fiber intake of 20 to 30 grams. Adequate fiber helps with proper bowel function. If you were to eat 1 cup of bran cereal, 1/2 cup of carrots, 1/2 cup of kidney beans, a medium-sized pear, and a medium-sized apple together in 1 day, you would get about 30 grams of fiber.

No more than 30 percent of calories, on average, from fat per day, with less than 10 percent of calories from saturated fat (such as fat from meat, butter, and eggs). Limiting fat to these levels reduces your risk for heart disease and may help you lose weight. In addition, you should limit the amount of cholesterol in your diet. Cholesterol is a fat-like substance found in animal products such as meat and eggs. Your diet should include no more than 300 milligrams of cholesterol per day (one egg contains about 215 milligrams of cholesterol, and 3.5 ounces of cooked hamburger contain 100 milligrams of cholesterol).

At least 8 to 10 glasses, 8 ounces each, of water or water-based beverages, per day. You need more water if you exercise a lot.

Types of Diets

Fixed-menu diet. A fixed-menu diet provides a list of all the foods you will eat. This kind of diet can be easy to follow because the foods are selected for you. But, you get very few different food choices which may make the diet boring and hard to follow away from home. In addition, fixed-menu diets do not teach the food selection skills necessary for keeping weight off. If you start with a fixed-menu diet, you should switch eventually to a plan that helps you learn to make meal choices on your own, such as an exchange-type diet.

Exchange-type diet. An exchange-type diet is a meal plan with a set number of servings from each of several food groups. Within each group, foods are about equal in calories and can be interchanged as you wish. For example, the "starch" category could include one slice of bread or 1/2 cup of oatmeal; each is about equal in nutritional value and calories. If your meal plan calls for two starch choices at breakfast, you could choose to eat two slices of bread, or one slice of bread and 1/2 cup of oatmeal. With the exchange-type diet plans, you have more day-to-day variety and you can easily follow the diet away from home. The most important advantage is that exchange-type diet plans teach the food selection skills you need to keep your weight off.

Prepackaged-meal diet. These diets require you to buy prepackaged meals. Such meals may help you learn appropriate portion sizes. However, they can be costly. Before beginning this type of program, find out whether you will need to buy the meals and how much the meals cost. You should also find out whether the program will teach you how to select and prepare food, skills that are needed to sustain weight loss. Formula diet. Formula diets are weight-loss plans that replace one or more meals with a liquid formula. Most formula diets are balanced diets containing a mix of protein, carbohydrate, and usually a small amount of fat. Formula diets are usually sold as liquid or a powder to be mixed with liquid. Although formula diets are easy to use and do promote short-term weight loss, most people regain the weight as soon as they stop using the formula. In addition, formula diets do not teach you how to make healthy food choices, a necessary skill for keeping your weight off.

Questionable diets. You should avoid any diet that suggests you eat a certain nutrient, food, or combination of foods to promote easy weight loss. Some of these diets may work in the short term because they are low in calories. However, they are often not well balanced and may cause nutrient deficiencies. In addition, they do not teach eating habits that are important for long-term weight management.

Flexible diets. Some programs or books suggest monitoring fat only, calories only, or a combination of the two, with the individual making the choice of both the type and amount of food eaten. This flexible type of approach works well for many people, and teaches them how to control what they eat. One drawback of flexible diets is that some don't consider the total diet. For example, programs that monitor fat only often allow people to take in unlimited amounts of excess calories from sugars, and therefore don't lead to weight loss.

It is important to choose an eating plan that you can live with. The plan should also teach you how to select and prepare healthy foods, as well as how to maintain your new weight. Remember that many people tend to regain lost weight. Eating a healthful and nutritious diet to maintain your new weight, combined with regular physical activity, helps to prevent weight regain.

Physical Activity

Regular physical activity is important to help you lose weight and build an overall healthy lifestyle. Physical activity increases the number of calories your body uses and promotes the loss of body fat instead of muscle and other nonfat tissue. Research shows that people who include physical activity in their weight-loss programs are more likely to keep their weight off than people who only change their diet. In addition to promoting weight control, physical activity improves your strength and flexibility, lowers your risk of heart disease, helps control blood pressure and diabetes, can promote a sense of well-being, and can decrease stress.

Any type of physical activity you choose to do—vigorous activities such as running or aerobic dancing or moderate-intensity activities such as walking or household work—will increase the number of calories your body uses. The key to successful weight control and improved overall health is making physical activity a part of your daily life. For the greatest overall health benefits, experts recommend that you do 20 to 30 minutes of vigorous physical activity three or more times a week and some type of muscle strengthening activity, such as weight resistance, and stretching at least twice a week. However, if you are unable to do this level of activity, you can improve your health by performing 30 minutes or more of moderate-intensity physical activity over the course of a day, at least five times a week. When including physical activity in your weight-loss program, you should choose a variety of activities that can be done regularly and are enjoyable for you. Also, if you have not been physically active, you should see your doctor before you start, especially if you are older than 40 years of age, very overweight, or have medical problems.

Behavior Change

Behavior change focuses on learning eating and physical activity behaviors that will help you lose weight and keep it off. The first step is to look at your eating and physical activity habits, thus uncovering behaviors (such as television watching) that lead you to overeat or be inactive. Next you'll need to learn how to change those behaviors.

Getting support from others is a good way to help you maintain your new eating and physical activity habits. Changing your eating and physical activity behaviors increases your chances of losing weight and keeping it off. For additional information on behavior change, you may wish to ask a weight-loss counselor or refer to books on this topic, which are available in local libraries.

What Works for You?

A variety of options exist to help you lose weight and keep it off. The key to successful weight loss is making changes in your eating and physical activity habits that you will be able to maintain for the rest of your life.

Depression

Everyone gets sad at times. But for those with depression, bad feelings come often. And these feelings get in the way of every day life.

About 12% of women in the U.S. suffer from depression. (That's almost 2 times as many as men.) Many people don't know the signs of depression. So they suffer when they do not need to. The good news is that almost 80% of depressed people get better with treatment.

What is clinical depression?

Clinical depression is a common form of mental illness. Depression can get in the way of caring about things, getting tasks done, or enjoying life.

What are the three main types of clinical depression?

Major depression is a mood or loss of interest that lasts most of the day, and every day for at least 2 weeks or longer.

Dysthymia (dis-thy-me-uh) is mild, and constant. It last 2 years or longer and it has the same signs as depression, but is milder. It doesn't interfere with daily life.

ten comes back many times over the person's lifetime.

Bipolar or manic depression involves mood swings between depression and mania.

What causes depression?

Medical illness
Losing someone you love
Stressful event

Drugs or alcohol
Family history of depression
Environmental factors
Chemical imbalance in the brain

What are the signs of depression?

Sadness, feeling "empty" a lot of the time
Loss of interest or pleasure in every day life
No interest in eating and losing weight; or overeating and gaining weight
Sleeping too much or too little, waking very early in the morning
Low energy, tired, feeling "slowed down"
Feeling restless, easily irritated, or crying a lot
Feeling guilty, worthless, helpless, hopeless, expecting the worst
Trouble staying focused, remembering, or making decisions
Thinking of death or suicide or trying to commit suicide

How can I tell if I am depressed?

A person is clinically depressed if he or she has five or more of these symptoms and has not been acting normal for most days during the same two-week period.

What are the signs of mania?

Unusually "high" mood
Easily irritated
Unable to go to sleep night after night
Grand notions (wild plans or ideas)

Talking too much
Racing thoughts
Increased activity, including sexual activity
Much more energy than usual
Poor judgment that leads to taking risks
Doing things that are not appropriate with or around other people

How is depression treated?

Depression is usually treated with both medicine (antidepressants) and counseling (talk therapy).

When taking your medicine, keep in mind...

You should take medicine for at least 4 to 6 months for it to work.

Anyone taking medicine for depression should be watched closely by a doctor.

Tell your doctor about other medicines you are taking. Many medicines interfere with antidepressants.

Caring for the Aging

When you think of family, your loved ones come to mind—a spouse, children, parents, grandparents, perhaps an aunt or uncle, or even someone special whom you consider "family." And, if you're lucky, these people are with you today, sharing in and contributing to fulfilling family life.

According to statistics, there's a good chance you will be enjoying their company for many years to come. Thanks to healthier lifestyles, advances in medicine and improved living conditions, the average life expectancy of a man today is 72, and it's 79 for a woman.

But with individuals living longer, the role of many adults has changed. Even if your loved ones are self-sufficient today, there is no guarantee their independent lifestyle and good physical health will continue. Eventually you may have the responsibility of arranging for their care. No one likes to think about the consequences of growing old, so this isn't an easy subject to bring up. But if you prepare and make plans now, you can lessen the stress and guilt during a crisis situation.

For starters, take a good look at your loved one's financial picture.

Explain that, not only do you want him to be comfortable in his retirement years, but you also want to arrange for his assets to be transferred according to his wishes upon his death. Talk with your loved one about his intentions, and include other family members in these discussions. Be direct and honest. Tell him your concerns, listen to his. That way if the time ever comes when your loved one cannot participate in the decision making, you'll know you are not acting alone, but carrying out his wishes.

Living Arrangements and Care Options.

When discussing who will provide continuous daily care for your loved one, you can choose from these general categories:

Independent living. Your loved one stays in his own home or rents an apartment and provides for himself. You oversee the situation and offer assistance and guidance when necessary.

Assisted-living community.

Your loved one lives independently in a facility that provides some additional support, such as light housekeeping, adult day services.

A community-based group program helps meet the needs of your loved one through an individualized plan of care. Such programs provide a structured comprehensive program in a protective setting for a part of each day, for example, while you're at work.

or daily meals. The facility may or may not have a nursing care option available for residents who become ill.

Home care.

You become responsible for seeing that a loved one's needs are met around the clock. You can move in with your loved one, move your loved one into your home, and, if necessary, either hire home health care professionals or become the sole caregiver yourself.

An intermediate care or skilled care facility, such as a nursing home.

These facilities are designed for people who need continuous, professional care at some level. Ask doctors, hospital discharge planners, social workers and friends for suggestions. You can also obtain a catalog of nursing homes from your state department of health or state agency on aging.

Discuss with your loved one what might happen if you can't maintain the level of care needed for him at home. Often people dread the idea of nursing homes and hospitals, but they may become necessary. On the other hand, these options may be out of financial reach so all other options must be exhausted first. Remind your loved one that the final decisions will depend largely on his health and finances at the time. Explain that you will try to carry out his preferences, but don't make promises you may not be able to keep.

Is Home Care the Answer?

If you think that home care may be the best alternative for your loved one, consider the following factors:

Physical and mental health.

Even if your loved one is in good health now, chronic and accelerating illnesses often accompany advancing age, and his state of health may change quickly. Such changes may dictate the type and level of care needed. Can your loved one manage routine chores and necessary tasks.

How much care will your loved one be able to pay for? How complex will that care be? Will they need custodial or skilled care? Are you prepared to subsidize their expenses? You may think your loved one has adequate financial reserves now, but those funds could be depleted if he lives another 15 years or more or comes down with a serious illness. Long-term care is expensive, whether you deliver the care or place your loved one in a nursing home.

Depending on where you live, home care can cost up to $35,000 a year and nursing home care can cost more than $55,000 a year.

Cooking, shopping, house and yard work and managing their finances? The more they can do for themselves, the greater their choices will be.

Your own family arrangement.

If you are married, your partner's feelings about the possibility of your becoming the care provider should be considered. And don't forget your children, especially if they still live at home. If there are disagreements, counseling might be a nonthreatening way to let all family members speak their minds. Family support.

The family unit is a major support system. Do you have family—or close friends—willing to share in the care giving or to lend financial or moral support? If so, accept help if they offer—and don't be afraid to ask for assistance.

Community services.

If you plan to assume complete responsibility for your loved one, be sure to check out community support services. Caretaker burnout can be avoided if you make good use of services from the beginning. To find out what's available, start with your local Area Agency on Aging or call the social services office at a local hospital. Some possibilities:

Hire a housecleaning or yard service.

Find a transportation volunteer through your church or local senior service organizations to drive your loved one to medical appointments or deliver groceries and prescriptions.

Use a meal service such as Meals on Wheels.

Enlist the services of a visiting nurse or a home health aide.

Inquire about senior center information and referral resources and adult day service facilities.

Contact the local chapters of associations, such as the Arthritis Foundation, the Alzheimer's Association, YMCA, American Red Cross and Veteran's Administration. They're often pipelines to the services available in your community.

Be good to yourself. Don't be a martyr—ask family and friends to help out. Consider joining a support group.

Making the Transition

Change is difficult for everyone, especially for the elderly, who may feel they already have lost control over much of their lives. If a new living arrangement involves uprooting a loved one to another city or town, he will need a considerate and caring transition. It helps to include him in the decision. If you are caring for your loved one long-distance, you may want to use the services of a geriatric care manager. For a fee, trained professionals provide a variety of services, such as helping to choose a health care facility, evaluating and monitoring care, and helping with activities of daily living.

Preparing Your Home

If you've decided care in your home is appropriate, you'll probably need to make some changes around the house. Changes can be as complex as adding another bathroom or converting a first-floor den into a bedroom or as simple as attaching a safety rail to the shower stall or having an amplified receiver installed on the telephone. Here are a few examples to get you started thinking:

Install a help alert system.

Remove clutter, sharp objects and throw rugs.

Place a flashlight by the bed.

Install nonskid strips in showers and bathtubs.

Install night-lights in halls and bathrooms.

Install railings next to all stairways and steps.

Set the hot water heater to a lower temperature.

Take a certified CPR course. In addition, you'll want to make your loved one feel welcome in your home by displaying his favorite possessions—particularly mementos and photographs—in plain sight.

Adjustment Strategies

Most people picture a loved one, particularly a spouse or parent, as eternally strong and capable. It's as hard for you to adjust to a loved one's physical decline as it is for him. Here are some ways to help both of you:

Make routines easy-to-follow, and try to stick to a schedule.

Good grooming is essential to your loved one's physical and emotional well-being. Include hair, nail, skin and dental care in your daily routine.

Make sure eyewear prescriptions are up-to-date. If your loved one's sight is failing, provide good lighting; a magnifying glass; large-print editions of books, newspapers and magazines; and other low-vision aids.

Ask how your loved one feels on a daily basis, and keep notes for the doctor.

Arrange regular dental checkups.

Consult your loved one's physician about dietary needs. Disease and medication can affect dietary requirements as much as age. If allowed, try to provide a variety of foods.

But don't forget to include your loved one's favorites. Also, make sure you serve food that can easily be chewed, cut up in manageable pieces or pureed, if necessary.

Maintaining Dignity

It's important that your loved one maintain a sense of personal dignity. Try to demonstrate respect with the following suggestions:

Be patient and calm.

If a loved one has difficulty hearing, speak slightly slower and use a lower pitch. Use simple, short sentences, and let your loved one see your face and expressions when speaking. Repeat and clarify when necessary-without being patronizing.

Make short, simple lists of daily activities and encourage your loved one to contribute.

Check off completed items each day.

No matter how helpless a loved one appears, don't reverse roles.

Treating a loved one like a child can crush any remaining feelings of dignity and independence.

Calmly discuss all plans and decisions.

Be positive and firm, and avoid emotional outbursts that only upset both of you.

Explain that you need your loved one's understanding and cooperation. If you reach an impasse, consult with a third party such as a care manager, doctor or member of the clergy.

Respect your loved one's religious or spiritual beliefs.

Help your loved one remain active and alert.

Encourage reading, hobbies and helping out around the house, if physically able. Welcome visitors and encourage your loved one to continue to participate in groups, clubs and organizations, if possible.

Caring for an aging loved one may be not only the most practical choice in your situation, but also the most rewarding.

Home care offers an opportunity to demonstrate your love and commitment. Sometimes unresolved issues in your relationship may come to the surface. It may be helpful to have a professional (a case manager, social worker, counselor or support group) assist you in working through these difficult times. Home care may not always be the easiest arrangement. But for those who approach it with a realistic attitude, caring for a loved one in a time of need can be a gratifying experience.

Growing Up Drug–Free

Bad habits can start early

The anti-drug education our children are getting in school today only begins to counter the street-level "education" they pick up from their peers and popular culture. Our children often learn how to use new media faster than we do, and they receive news and entertainment not only from movies and TV, but from video cassettes, CDs, billboards, magazines targeted to children, websites, and chat rooms—information sources and formats that didn't even exist a generation ago. Drug references can reach them in unexpected places, such as magazine ads and clothing-store dressing rooms where music is piped in. Even though these sights and sounds are not usually promoting drug use, they can reinforce a child's impression that use is "normal"—a standard, even expected, part of growing up.

Unfortunately, the perception that drugs are a normal rite of passage has become common even among children in their preteen years. Many parents of nine-to-twelve year-olds would be shocked to learn how plentiful—and often free—drugs are in their children's world. The average age at which teens start using tobacco is a little past 12 years old. The average age at which they start drinking alcohol is almost 13. And the average age at which they start smoking marijuana is 14. Although the majority of young people do not use these substances, some children are using at even younger ages than these.

It could be your child

These statistics are so startling that it's tempting to think, "My child would never do anything so risky at that age." But believing that is risky in itself. Studies show that many more teens report being offered drugs—and using them—than their parents are willing to believe. When polled, the number of parents who thought their children had tried marijuana—about 20%—represented only one-half the number of teens who said they had actually tried.

Although keeping a child drug-free through these trying years is a great challenge to a parent, no one is in a better position than you to meet this challenge. A study published in the Journal of the American Medical Association found that teenagers who reported feeling close to their families were the least likely to engage in any of the risky behaviors studied, which included drinking and smoking marijuana or cigarettes. This finding supports what a majority of parents believe: that they can teach their children to view drugs as a serious concern and that they can influence their children's decisions about whether or not to use drugs.

This information will help you guide your preschool-to-high school-age children as they form attitudes about drug use. It provides answers to children's questions.

How to carry on a continuing dialogue with your children on the subject of drugs. Talking frequently is essential, and it's important to be clear; research found that although nine out of ten parents questioned said that in the past year they had talked to their teens about drugs, only two-thirds of the teens agreed.

Why occasional alcohol, tobacco or other drug use is a serious matter. Even a child who may get drunk or high on cocaine less than once a month can suffer serious consequences, such as flunking an important test, having a car accident, or a heart attack.

How to educate ourselves. To talk to our children persuasively, we need to have as much information as they do. This information provides a working knowledge of common drugs—their effects on the mind and body, the symptoms of their use, the latest drug slang, and methods of drug use now in vogue.

The teen years can be trying for families. It is not always easy to communicate with those you love. But the stakes are high. If teens can navigate these years without drinking, smoking, or taking drugs, chances are that they won't use or abuse these substances as adults. Your influence early on can spare your child the negative experiences associated with illegal drug use, and even save your child's life.

Why you shouldn't allow your children to smoke marijuana

Some parents who saw marijuana being widely used in their youth have wondered, "Is marijuana really so bad for my child?" The answer is an emphatic "yes," and parents should familiarize themselves with these reasons:

Marijuana is illegal. Marijuana now exists in forms that are stronger—with higher levels of THC, the psychoactive ingredient—than in the 1960s.
Studies show that someone who smokes five joints a week may be taking in as many cancer-causing chemicals as someone who smokes a full pack of cigarettes every day.

Hanging around users of marijuana often means being exposed not only to other drugs later on, but also to a lifestyle that can include trouble in school, engaging in sexual activity while young, unintended pregnancy, difficulties with the law, and other problems.

Marijuana use can slow down reaction time and distort perceptions. This can interfere with athletic performance, decrease a sense of danger, and increase risk of injury.

Regular marijuana users can lose the ability to concentrate that is needed to master important academic skills, and they can experience short-term memory loss. Habitual marijuana users tend to do worse in school and are much more likely to drop out altogether.
Teens who rely on marijuana as a chemical crutch and refuse to face the challenges of growing up never learn the emotional, psychological, and social lessons of adolescence.
The research is not complete on the effects of marijuana on the developing brain and body.

Planning for togetherness

Sometimes it's frustrating how few chances there are to have conversations about drugs with our children. In our busy culture, with families juggling the multiple demands of work, school, after-school activities, and religious and social commitments, it can be a challenge for parents and children to be in the same place at the same time. To ensure that you have regular get togethers with your children, try to schedule:

Family meetings.
Held once a week at a mutually-agreed-upon time, family meetings provide a forum for discussing triumphs, grievances, projects, questions about discipline, and any topic of concern to a family member. Ground rules help. Everyone gets a

chance to talk; one person talks at a time without interruption; everyone listens, and only positive, constructive feedback is allowed. To get resistant children to join in, combine the get-together with incentives such as post-meeting pizza or assign them important roles such as recording secretary or rule enforcer.

Regular parent-child rituals.

These eliminate the need for constant planning and rearranging. Perhaps you can take the long way home from school once a week and get ice cream or make a weekly visit to the library together. Even a few minutes of conversation while you're cleaning up after dinner or right before bedtime can help the family catch up and establish the open communication that is essential to raising drug-free children.

Making your position clear

When it comes to dangerous substances like alcohol, tobacco, and other drugs, don't assume that your children know where you stand. **They want you to talk to them about drugs. State your position clearly; if you're ambiguous, children may be tempted to use.** Tell your children that you forbid them to use alcohol, tobacco, and drugs because you love them. (Don't be afraid to pull out all the emotional stops. You can say, "If you took drugs it would break my heart.") Make it clear that this rule holds true even at other people's houses.

Will your child listen? Most likely. According to research, when a child decides whether or not to use alcohol, tobacco, and other drugs, a crucial consideration is "What will my parents think?"

Also discuss the consequences of breaking the rules—what the punishment will be and how it will be carried out. Consequences must go hand-in-hand with limits so that your child understands that there's a predictable outcome to his choosing a particular course of action. **The consequences you select should be reasonable and related to the violation.** For example, if you catch your son smoking, you might "ground" him, restricting his social activities for two weeks. You could then use this time to show him how concerned you are about the serious health consequences of his smoking, and about the possibility that he'll become addicted, by having him study articles, books, or video tapes on the subject.

Whatever punishment you settle on shouldn't involve new penalties that you didn't discuss before the rule was broken—this wouldn't be fair. Nor should you issue empty threats ("Your father will kill you when he gets home!"). It's understandable that you'd be angry when house rules are broken, and sharing your feelings of anger, disappointment, or sadness can have a powerfully motivating effect on your child. Since we're all more inclined to say things we don't mean when we're upset, it's best to cool off enough to discuss consequences in a matter-of-fact way.

Contrary to some parents' fears, your strict rules won't alienate your children. They *want* you to show you care enough to lay down the law and to go to the trouble of enforcing it. Rules about what's acceptable, from curfews to insisting that they call in to tell you where they are, make children feel loved and secure.

Rules about drugs also give them reasons to fall back on when they feel tempted to make bad decisions. A recent poll showed that drugs are the number-one concern of young people today. Even when they appear nonchalant, our children need and want parental guidance. It does not have to be preachy. You will know best when it is more effective to use an authoritarian tone or a gentler approach.

Always let your children know how happy you are that they respect the rules of the household by praising them. **Emphasize the things your children do right instead of focusing on what's wrong.** When parents are quicker to praise than to criticize, children learn to feel good about themselves, and they develop the self-confidence to trust their own judgment.

What your own alcohol, tobacco, and drug use tells your children

Drinking alcohol is one of the accepted practices of adulthood. It is legal for adults to have wine with dinner, beer at the end of a long week, or cocktails at a dinner party. But drinking to the point of losing control sends the wrong message to children, as does reaching for a drink to remedy unhappiness or tension.

Although it is legal for adults to smoke cigarettes, the negative impact tobacco has on a smoker's health is well documented. If a child asks his parents why they smoke, they may explain that when they began, people didn't understand how unhealthy smoking is and that once a smoker starts, it's very hard to stop. Young people can avoid making the same mistake their parents did by never starting and risking addiction.

When parents smoke marijuana or use other illegal drugs, they compromise not only their children's sense of security and safety, but the children's developing moral codes as well. If you use illegal drugs, it is self-deluding to imagine that your children won't eventually find out. When they do, your parental credibility and authority will go out the window. If their parents—their closest and most important role models—don't respect the law, then why should they? Parents who abuse alcohol or other drugs should seek professional help. This help is available at treatment centers and from support groups such as Alcoholics Anonymous and Narcotics Anonymous. Their children also may benefit from professional counseling and support from groups such as Families Anonymous, Al-Anon, and Nar-Anon.

What to say when your child asks, "Did you ever use drugs?"

Among the most common drug-related questions asked of parents is "Did you ever use drugs?" Unless the answer is "no," it's difficult to know what to say because nearly all parents who used drugs don't want their children to do the same thing. Is this hypocritical? No. We all want the best for our children, and we understand the hazards of drug use better than we did when we were their age and thought we were invincible. To guide our children's decisions about drugs, we can now draw on credible real-life examples of friends who had trouble as a result of their drug use: the neighbor who caused a fatal car crash while high; the family member who got addicted; the teen who used marijuana for years, lost interest in school, and never really learned how to deal with adult life and its stresses.

Some parents who used drugs in the past choose to lie about it, but they risk losing their credibility if their children discover the truth. Many experts recommend that when a child asks this question, the response should be honest.

This doesn't mean that parents need to recount every moment of their experiences. As in conversations about sex, some details should remain private, and you should avoid providing more information than is actually sought by your child. Ask clarifying questions to make sure you understand exactly why and what a child is asking before answering questions about your past drug use, and limit your response to that information.

This discussion provides a good opportunity for parents to speak frankly about what attracted them to drugs, why drugs are dangerous, and why they want their children to avoid making the same mistake. There's no perfect way to get this message across, only approaches that seem more fitting than others.

How grandparents can help raise drug-free children

Grandparents play a special part in a child's life and, unlike parents, grandparents have had years to prepare for their role. They've been through the ups and downs of child-rearing and bring a calmer, more seasoned approach to their interactions with their grandchildren. They, as well as other extended family members, can serve as stable, mature role models, especially if they need to step in to assume some of the responsibilities of the child's parents.

These important elders have one advantage over parents: Their relationships with their grandchildren are less complicated, less judgmental, and less tied to day-to-day stresses. Grandparents can use their positions of trust and intimacy to reinforce the same lessons in self-respect and healthy living that children are learning from their parents. When grandparents show concern with questions like "Has anyone ever tried to sell you drugs?" or "Why are your eyes so red?" they may be more likely to hear honest answers—especially if they indicate that they are willing to listen in confidence, and will not be quick to judge or punish. Their grandchildren may be less defensive and more likely to listen closely to their advice about avoiding drugs. Grandparents can also help reinforce positive messages and praise their grandchildren when they do well.

Why a child uses drugs

Understandably, some parents of drug users think that their child might have been pressured into taking drugs by peers or drug dealers. But children say they choose to use drugs because they want to:

relieve boredom
feel good
forget their troubles and relax
have fun
satisfy their curiosity
take risks
ease their pain
feel grown-up
show their independence
belong to a specific group
look cool

Rather than being influenced by new friends whose habits they adopt, children and teens often switch peer groups so they can hang around with others who have made the same lifestyle choices.

Parents know their children best and are therefore in the best position to suggest healthy alternatives to doing drugs. Sports, clubs, music lessons, community service projects, and after-school activities not only keep children and teens active and interested, but also bring them closer to parents who can attend games and performances. To develop a positive sense of independence, you could encourage babysitting or tutoring. For a taste of risk-taking, suggest rock-climbing, karate, or camping.

What our culture tells children about drugs

Unfortunately, the fashions and fads that thrive in our culture are sometimes the ones with the most shock value. Children today are surrounded by subtle and overt messages telling them what is "good" about alcohol, tobacco, and drugs. Your children may see TV characters living in wealth and splendor off drug money, may stumble onto a website urging legalization of marijuana, may see their favorite movie stars smoking in their latest films, or may hear songs describing the thrill of making love while high.

To combat these impressions, put your television and computer in a communal area so you can keep tabs on what your children are seeing. Sit down with them when they watch TV. Explore the Internet with them to get a feel for what they like. Anything disturbing can be turned into a "teachable moment." You may want to set guidelines for which TV shows, films, and websites are appropriate for your child. (You also may want to reassure children that the world is not as bleak as it appears in the news, which focuses heavily on society's problems.)

In the same way, familiarize yourself with your children's favorite radio stations, CDs, and tapes. According to a recent survey, most teenagers consider listening to music their favorite non-school activity and, on average, devote three to four hours to it every day. Since many of the songs they hear make drug use sound inviting and free of consequences, you'll want to combat this impression with your own clear position.

Signs that your child might be using drugs

Since mood swings and unpredictable behavior are frequent occurrences for pre-teens and teenagers, parents may find it difficult to spot signs of alcohol and drug abuse. But if your child starts to exhibit one or more of these signs (which apply equally to sons and daughters), drug abuse may be at the heart of the problem:
She's withdrawn, depressed, tired, and careless about personal grooming.
He's hostile and uncooperative; he frequently breaks curfews.
Her relationships with family members have deteriorated.
He's hanging around with a new group of friends.
Her grades have slipped, and her school attendance is irregular.
He's lost interest in hobbies, sports, and other favorite activities.
Her eating or sleeping patterns have changed; she's up at night and sleeps during the day.
He has a hard time concentrating.
Her eyes are red-rimmed and/or her nose is runny in the absence of a cold.
Household money has been disappearing.
The presence of pipes, rolling papers, small medicine bottles, eye drops, or butane lighters in your home signal that your child may be using drugs. Other clues include homemade pipes and bongs (pipes that use water as a filter) made from soda cans or plastic beverage containers. If any of these indicators show up, parents should start discussing what steps to take so they can present a united front. They may also want to seek other family members' impressions.

Acting on your suspicions

If you suspect that your child is using drugs, you should voice your suspicions openly—avoiding direct accusations—when he or she is sober or straight and you're calm.

This may mean waiting until the next day if he comes home drunk from a party, or if her room reeks of marijuana. Ask about what's been going on—in school and out—and discuss how to avoid using drugs and alcohol in the future. If you encounter reluctance to talk, enlist the aid of your child's school guidance counselor, family physician, or a local drug treatment referral and assessment center—they may get a better response. Also explore what could be going on in your child's emotional or social life that might prompt drug use.

Taking the time to discuss the problem openly without turning away is an important first step on the road to recovery. It shows that your child's well-being is crucial to you and that you still love him, although you hate what he's doing to himself. But you should also show your love by being firm and enforcing whatever discipline your family has agreed upon for violating house rules. You should go over ways to regain the family's trust such as calling in, spending evenings at home, and improving grades.

Even in the face of mounting evidence, parents often have a hard time acknowledging that their child has an alcohol, tobacco, or drug problem. Anger, resentment, guilt, and a sense of failure are all common reactions, but it is important to avoid self-blame. Drug abuse occurs in families of all economic and social backgrounds, in happy and unhappy homes alike. Most important is that the faster you act, the sooner your child can start to become well again.

Addiction

No one who begins to use drugs thinks he or she will become addicted. Addiction is a disease characterized by compulsive drug-seeking behavior regardless of the consequences. Research conducted by the National Institute on Drug Abuse clearly shows that virtually all drugs that are abused have a profound effect on the brain. Prolonged use of many drugs including cocaine, heroin, marijuana and amphetamines can change the brain in fundamental and long-lasting ways, resulting in drug craving and addiction.

If and when a drug abuser becomes addicted depends on the individual.

Research shows that children who use alcohol and tobacco are more likely to use marijuana than children who do not use these substances. Children who use marijuana are more likely to use other addictive drugs. Certain genetic, social, and environmental risk factors make it more likely that certain individuals will become addicted to alcohol, tobacco, and other drugs. These include:

children of alcoholics who, according to several studies, may have inherited genes that make them more prone to addiction, and who may have had more stressful upbringings;

sensation-seekers who may like the novelty of feeling drunk or high;
children with psychological problems, such as conduct disorders, who self-medicate to feel better;
children with learning disabilities, and others who find it difficult to fit in or become frustrated learning;
children of poverty who lack access to opportunities to succeed and to resources when they're in trouble.
The more risk factors children have, the greater their vulnerability. And everyone has a different ability to tolerate drugs and alcohol—what if your child's tolerance is very low?
Regardless of how "cool" drugs may look, there is nothing glamorous about the reality of addiction, a miserable experience for the addict and everyone around him. Addiction causes an all-consuming craving for drugs, leading an otherwise responsible, caring person to destroy relationships, work, and family life.

Finding the right treatment

Certified drug and alcohol counselors work with families to find the program best suited to a child's needs. To find a good certified counselor you can consult your child's doctor, other parents whose children have been treated for drug abuse, the local hospital, a school social worker, the school district's substance abuse coordinator, or the county mental health society.

Addiction is a treatable disease

The success of any treatment approach depends on a variety of factors such as the child's temperament and willingness to change, and the extent and frequency of use. Drug addiction is now understood to be a chronic, relapsing disease. It is not surprising, then, that parents may have to make a number of attempts at intervention before their child can remain drug-free, and they should not despair if their first try does not produce long-lasting results. Even if it is not apparent at the time, each step brings the child closer to being healthy.

Staying Active

Staying active as you age helps you remain healthy, live longer and feel better.

More older people than ever before are involved in exercise and sports. They've learned that being physically fit doesn't have to mean aching muscles from workouts and hard-to-maintain exercise schedules. Many people are getting their exercise in active pastimes such as biking, skiing and tennis. Others prefer less active recreation such as walking, gardening or golf.

All are finding relaxation and fun while they secure a healthy future. Exercise helps you feel better because it improves your health. Orthopedic surgeons say that by spending a little time each day in some type of physical activity, you can enjoy these significant benefits:

longer, healthier life
stronger bones
reduced joint and muscle pain
improved mobility and balance
lower risk of falls and serious injuries like hip fractures
slower loss of muscle mass
People are living longer these days and
their quality of life depends on being healthy and remaining independent. Staying active can lower your risk for many common diseases, relieve the pain of arthritis and help you to recover faster when you do get sick.

Stay active and safe

While it's important to stay active, it's also important to play it safe. As more older people engage in physical activities, sports-related injuries are increasing. This is especially true for those who ride bicycles, ski, lift weights and use exercise machines.
By getting regular exercise-and doing it safely-you can enjoy a healthier life.

Seven tips to prevent injury

When you exercise, orthopedic surgeons recommend that you follow these tips:

Always wear appropriate safety gear. If YOU bike, always wear a bike helmet. Wear the appropriate shoes for each sport.

Warm-up before you exercise. That could be a moderate activity such as walking at your normal pace, while emphasizing your arm movements.

Exercise for at least 30 minutes a day. You can break this into shorter periods of 10 or 15 minutes during the day.

Follow the 10 percent rule. Never increase your program (i.e., walking or running distance or amount of weight lifted) more than 10 percent a week.

Try not to do the exact same routine two days in a row. Walk, swim, play tennis or lift weights. This works different muscles and keeps exercise more interesting.

When working out with exercise equipment, read instructions carefully and, if needed, ask someone qualified to help you. Check treadmills or other exercise equipment to be sure they are in good working order. If You are new to weight training, make sure you get proper information before you begin.

Stop exercising if you experience severe pain or swelling. Discomfort that persists should always be evaluated.

There are lots of ways to enhance your life as you age-and staying fit is one of the most important.

Understanding Prostate Changes:
A Health Guide for All Men

The prostate, scarcely noticed by the public a decade ago, is now in the limelight, featured in thousands of reports in the general press and in medical journals. Why has interest soared? There are several reasons.

Famous figures such as Harry Belafonte, Bob Dole, and Norman Schwartzkopf have gone public after being struck by prostate cancer. By doing that, they have spurred interest in the small gland and rallied support for increased research and better treatment choices.

Also, more men are living to older ages-when prostate enlargement is common and prostate cancer becomes more likely-and huge numbers of previously unsuspected, symptom-free prostate cancers are being identified through simple blood-screening tests.

Despite all the attention, however, issues surrounding the prostate, and prostate cancer in particular, are immersed in uncertainty. It is not known, for instance, if the potential benefits of prostate cancer screening outweigh the risks, if surgery is better than radiation, or if treatment is better than no treatment in some cases.

Because of these uncertainties, doctors and medical organizations offer conflicting advice for men who are weighing their options. As a result, men often find themselves confused about what to do next.

By providing some insight into the prostate and prostate disorders, this information aims to help you consult knowledgeably with your doctor in order to weigh your alternatives.

The **prostate gland**, a key part of the male reproductive system, is linked closely with the urinary system. It is a small gland that secretes much of the liquid portion of **semen**, the milky fluid that transports **sperm** through the **penis** when a man ejaculates.

The prostate is located just beneath the **bladder**, where **urine** is stored, and in front of the **rectum**. It encircles, like a donut, a section of the **urethra**. The urethra is the tube that carries urine front the bladder out through the penis. During **ejaculation**, semen is secreted by the prostate through small pores in the urethra's walls.

The prostate is made up of three lobes encased in an outer covering, or **capsule**. It is flanked on either side by the **seminal vesicles**, a pair of pouch-like glands that contribute secretions to the semen. Next to the seminal vesicles run the two **vas deferens**, tubes that carry sperm from the **testicles**. The testicles, in addition to manufacturing sperm, also produce **testosterone**, a male sex **hormone** that controls the prostate's growth and function.

The prostate usually is healthy in younger men. As a man grows older, however, the prostate gland frequently becomes a source of trouble. The three most common prostate problems are inflammation (**prostatitis**), prostate enlargement (**benign prostatic hyperplasia/BPH**), and **prostate cancer**.

I. Prostatitis

Prostatitis, or prostate inflammation, can cause difficult or painful urination that often is accompanied by a burning sensation, by a strong and frequent urge to urinate that often results in only small amounts of urine, and by pain in the lower back or abdomen.

The causes of prostatitis are unclear. Sometimes, it is the result of a bacterial infection. At other times, the cause is unknown. Occasionally, prostatitis is accompanied by chills and a high fever. When prostatitis is the result of a bacterial infection, it usually can be cleared up with antibiotics.

II. Benign Prostatic Hyperplasia (BPH)

Benign prostatic hvperplasia (BPH) is an enlarged prostate. **Benign** means non-cancerous and **hyperplasia** means excessive growth of tissue. BPH is the result of small noncancerous growths inside the prostate. It is not known what causes these growths, but they may be related to hormone changes that occur with aging. By age 60, more than half of all American men have **microscopic** signs of BPH, and by age 70, more than 40 percent will have enlargement that can he felt on physical examination.

The prostate normally starts out about the site of a walnut. By the time a man is age 40, the prostate may already have grown to the size of an apricot; by the age of 60, it may be as big as a lemon.

BPH, which usually does not affect sexual function, is a troublemaker because the prostate, as it enlarges, presses against the bladder and the urethra, blocking the flow of urine.

A man with BPH may find it difficult to initiate a urine than a dribble. He also may need to urinate frequently, or he may have a sudden, powerful large to urinate. Many men are forced to get up several times a night; others have an annoying feeling that the bladder is never completely empty.

Straining to empty the bladder can make matters worse; the bladder stretches, the bladder wall thickens and loses its elasticity, and the bladder muscles become less efficient. The pool of urine that collects in the bladder can foster urinary tract infections, and trying to force a urine strain can produce backpressure that eventually damages the **kidneys**. The kidneys are where urine is formed, as waste products are filtered from the blood.

BPH sometimes leads to problems. For instance, a completely blocked urethra is a medical emergency requiring immediate catheterization, a procedure in which a tube called a **catheter** is inserted through the penis into the bladder to allow urine to escape. Other serious potential complications of BPH include bladder stones and bleeding.

Diagnosing BPH

A detailed medical history focusing on the urinary tract—kidneys, **ureters** (the pair of tubes that carry urine from the kidneys to the bladder), the bladder, and the urethra—allows the doctor to identify **symptoms** and to evaluate the possibility of infection or other urinary problems.

The initial medical workup typically includes a physical exam called a **digital rectal examination (DRE)**, a **urinalysis** to check for infection or bleeding, and a blood test to measure kidney function. Some physicians may also check the amount of **prostate-specific antigen (PSA)**, using a **PSA test** to help rule out the likelihood of cancer. PSA is a protein that is produced by the cells of the prostate gland.

In addition, other tests may help a **urologist**—a doctor who specializes in disorders of the urinary tract and the male reproductive tract-to determine if BPH has affected the bladder or kidneys. These include tests that measure the speed of urine flow, pressure in the bladder during urination, and how much urine is left in the bladder after urinating.

Some other tests that are widely used, according to an expert panel sponsored by the United States Public Health Service (USPHS) practice guidelines, are expensive, sometimes risky, and, for most men, unnecessary. These include **cystoscopy**, in which the doctor inserts a viewing tube up the urethra to get a direct look at the bladder; an **x-ray** called a **urogram**, in which urine is made visible on an x-ray after dye is injected into a vein; and **ultrasound**, which obtains images of the kidneys and bladder after a probe is placed on the abdomen.

Treating BPH

About half of the men with BPH develop symptoms serious enough to warrant treatment. BPH cannot be cured, but its symptoms can be relieved by surgery or by drugs in many cases.

BPH does not necessarily grow worse. According to one review, mild to moderate symptoms worsened in only about 20 percent of the cases. They improved (without any specific treatment) in another 20 percent, and stayed about the same in the rest.

Men whose symptoms are mild often opt for an approach called **watchful waiting**. This means that they report for regular checkups and have further treatment only if and when their symptoms become too bothersome.

The USPHS Clinical Practice Guidelines call watchful waiting "an appropriate treatment strategy for the majority of patients." Men who choose watchful waiting should have regular, perhaps annual, checkups, including DREs and laboratory tests.

For those who choose watchful waiting, a number of simple steps may help to reduce bothersome symptoms. These include limiting fluid intake in the evening, especially beverages containing alcohol or caffeine, which can trigger the urge to urinate and can interfere with sleep; taking time to empty the bladder completely; and not allowing long intervals to pass without urinating.

Men monitoring prostate conditions should also be aware that certain medications they are taking for other ailments may make their symptoms worse. These include some over-the-counter cough and cold remedies, prescribed tranquilizers, antidepressants, and drugs to control high blood pressure. Switching to a different prescription may help.

Watchful waiting, of course, is not always enough for BPH, and surgery or drug therapy may be required. Here is a close look at both options:

BPH Surgery

Although the popularity of prostate surgery has diminished since drug therapy became available, operations for BPH remain the most common surgery performed on American men.

Several types of surgery can relieve the symptoms of an enlarged prostate. They are:

Transurethral Resection of the Prostate (TURP). This procedure accounts for more than 90 percent of all BPH surgeries. TURF relieves symptoms quickly, typically doubling the urinary flow within weeks.

Here is how the surgery is done. The patient is numbed from the waist down with an **anesthetic** injection known as a **spinal block**. The surgeon then inserts a slim fiber optic tube through the penis and up the urethra as far as the prostate. Using either a tiny blade or an electric loop, the surgeon pares away the urethras lining and bits of excess prostate tissue. Gradually the passageway is expanded.

A TURP patient is usually hospitalized for several days after surgery. During convalescence, a catheter remains in the bladder through the penis to drain out urine. By the time the patient leaves the hospital, he is usually able to urinate on his own.

The TURF procedure ordinarily does not pose the two main dangers generally linked to prostate surgery: **incontinence** (loss of urinary control) and problems with sexual function, especially **sexual impotence** (the inability to have an **erection**).

About 5 percent of men become partially incontinent after the TURF procedure although the incontinence sometimes clears up over time. In addition, some men develop scarring in the urethra that can block urination. As many as 10 percent will need repeat surgery because prostate tissue grows back.

About 5 percent of men become impotent after the TURF procedure. But TURF does not usually affect a man's ability to have an erection or an **orgasm**, since the nerves that control erection lie outside the prostate and are not touched by the operation. A more common side effect is a dry, or retrograde, ejaculation. It occurs after surgery when the neck of the bladder fails to close properly during ejaculation. The result is that semen spurts backward into the bladder rather than through the penis. Men who experience this side effect still have the sensation of an orgasm but are unable to father children.

Transurethral Incision of the Prostate (TUIP). This procedure is used on small prostate glands of 30 grams or less and is used far less frequently than TURF.

Like TURF, TUIP is performed by passing an instrument through the penis to reach the prostate. The difference is that a doctor makes only one or two small cuts to relieve pressure in the prostate rather than trimming away tissue. Like TURP, the procedure considerably increases the urine flow.

TUIP is an outpatient procedure with a low risk of **side effects**. Because of that, the USPHS, Clinical Practice Guidelines recommend that the technique be used more often.

Transurethral Needle Ablation (TUNA). This recently approved technique, which can be done with a local anesthetic on an outpatient basis, uses radio frequency energy delivered through needles to kill excess prostate tissue. A catheter that deploys the needles toward the obstructing prostate tissue is inserted into the urethra before the procedure begins. Some clinical studies have reported that TUNA improves the urine flow with minimal side effects when compared with other procedures.

Open Prostatectomy. The word "open" refers to the fact that a surgeon makes an incision to reach the prostate, instead of inserting an instrument through the urethra. Open prostatectomy may involve either a radical or a partial procedure. A **radical prostatectomy**, which removes the whole prostate, is done for cancer. The incision is made through either the lower abdomen or the **perineum**. **Partial prostatectomy**, which leaves the posterior portion of the prostate intact, is used to treat BPH. The incision for a partial prostatectomy is usually through the abdomen. Open prostatectomy once was the sole recourse for an enlarged prostate. Today it is used only on extremely large prostates, which represent about 5 percent of all cases.

BPH Drug Therapy

Millions of American men have chosen drugs over surgery since drug therapy for BPH made its debut in the early 1990s. Although regarded as less effective than surgery, drugs are also less invasive and usually free of major side effects.

There are two major classes of drugs: **alpha adrenergic blockers** and **finasteride**.

Alpha adrenergic blockers were originally used for the treatment of high blood pressure, to relax smooth muscles in blood vessel walls. In BPH, they relax the muscular portion of the prostate and the **bladder neck**. This allows urine to flow more freely. In the average patient, these drugs increase the rate of urine flow and reduce symptoms, often within days. Side effects include dizziness, fatigue, and headache.

Finasteride shrinks the prostate by blocking an **enzyme** that converts the male hormone testosterone into a more potent, growth-stimulating form. Some, but not all, studies show that taking finasteride for at least six months can increase urinary flow rate and reduce symptoms. It seems to work best for men who have greatly enlarged prostates. In a small percentage of men, the drug can affect sexual activity, decreasing a man's interest in sex, diminishing his ability to have an erection, and causing problems with ejaculation. It sometimes also reuses tenderness or swelling of the breasts. It may cause a drop in PSA levels. These side effects can be reversed by stopping the drug.

Some doctors think that combining the two types of drugs may produce better results.

Researchers are working to develop BPH treatments that are more effective and less traumatic, with fewer side effects. These include using laser surgery, powerful electric currents, and microwaves. Doctors have also tried to enlarge the urethra by inserting a balloon into it and inflating it with fluid, and by inserting a **stent** (a small metal coil) into the urethra to hold it open.

Choosing a Treatment for BPH

If a man has no serious complications such as the inability to urinate, kidney damage, frequent urinary tract infections, major bleeding through the urethra, or bladder stones, the best approach for treating BPH is not clear.

The USPHS Clinical Practice Guidelines advise doctors to leave treatment decisions to the patient, after a discussion of the benefits and side effects of each treatment option.

The options selected by an individual man are tied to his own preferences. For instance, some men want immediate relief and are willing to undergo surgery or embrace a drug regimen to get that relief. Some men also are eager to take drugs even if their only symptom is an elevated PSA level. Others are reluctant, often unwilling, to undergo surgery or to take pills daily for an extended period.

III. Evaluating Prostate Health

Digital Rectal Examination (DRE).

The standard technique for evaluating the health of the prostate is by physical examination called a digital rectal exam (DRE). Typically, a patient is asked to bend forward over a table while the doctor inserts a gloved and lubricated finger (called a digit in the medical community) into the patient's rectum. This allows the physician to feel the back portion of the prostate gland. In addition to gauging the gland's size, the doctor is able to evaluate its firmness and texture. The doctor looks for answers to some key questions: Has its usual rubbery feel changed? Are there any hard areas or lumps, which could signal a cancer? Has a growth spread beyond the prostate?

Prostate-Specific Antigen (PSA).

This is a substance produced by cells of the prostate gland. PSA circulates in the blood and can be detected and measured with a relatively simple blood test. When the gland enlarges, PSA levels rise. PSA levels can also rise if cancer develops.

Generally, doctors consider readings below 4 nanograms per milliliter (ng/ml) to be normal, scores between 4 and 10 to be slightly elevated, scores between 10 and 20 to be moderately elevated, and anything above that to be highly elevated. Most men with BPH have levels of 10 ng/ml or below.

However, many factors can influence PSA levels. Some prostate glands naturally produce more PSA than others. PSA scores also tend to increase with age. Another influence on PSA levels is race: PSA levels tend to be higher in African-Americans, and lower among Japanese, than in white Americans.
A variety of conditions can raise PSA levels temporarily. These include prostatitis, prostate **biopsy**, and transurethral prostate surgery.
Transrectal Ultrasound (TRUS).

This procedure uses a small probe that is inserted into the rectum. The probe emits and picks up high-frequency sound waves. The sound waves bounce off the prostate, producing a pattern that is converted into a video image. Areas of cancer produce a different pattern than healthy tissue. The value of a TRUS is strongly influenced by the quality of the equipment and the skill of the person operating it.

While ultrasound does not provide enough specific information to make it a good screening tool by itself, doctors find it useful as a follow-up to a suspicious DRE or PSA. TRUS is also used to guide biopsies in sampling abnormal areas of the prostate, to estimate the volume of the prostate for calculating PSA density, and to situate radiotherapy implants.

IV. Prostate Cancer
Like other cancers, prostate cancer is a disease of cells growing out of control. Spurred by changes in the genes, the glandular cells of the prostate multiply abnormally. These cancer cells may cross tissue barriers and may then spread throughout the body.

Compared with most cancers, prostate cancer tends to grow slowly. It may be decades from the time the earliest cell changes can be detected under a microscope until the cancer gets big enough to cause symptoms.

By age 50, one-third of American men have microscopic signs of prostate cancer, and by age 75, half to three-quarters of men's prostates will have cancerous changes. Most of these cancers either remain **latent**, producing no **signs** or symptoms, or they are so slow-growing, or **indolent**, that they never become a serious threat to health.

A much smaller number of men will actually be treated for prostate cancer. About 16 percent of American men will be diagnosed with prostate cancer during their lifetime; 8 percent will develop significant symptoms; and 3 percent will die of the disease.

The late 1980s saw a sharp hike in the number of cases being diagnosed. By 1997, the number of new cases of prostate cancer reached an estimated 209,000, more than double the 90,000 cases identified just 10 years earlier. However, recent statistics show that the incidence rate (the number of cases diagnosed per 100,000 men per year) has begun to decline.

Much of the dramatic surge in the detection of prostate cancer cases can be traced to the growing use of procedures and tests that, intentionally or not, reveal small, symptom-free cancers, many of which otherwise would have gone unnoticed.

Before the 1980s, prostate cancer usually was diagnosed either when it caused symptoms or during a digital rectal exam (DRE).

It was in the mid-1980s, when doctors began using the transurethral resection of the prostate (TURF) procedure to treat benign prostate enlargement, that small, even microscopic cancers began turning up in prostate tissue samples removed at surgery.

The number of prostate cancer diagnoses rose even faster in the late 1980s when doctors began to add the blood test for prostate-specific antigen (PSA) to regular checkups. A National Cancer Institute (NCI) study showed that doctors increased their use of the PSA test for men ages 65 or older-the age group most susceptible to prostate cancer-from 1,430 per 100,000 men in 1988 to 18,000 per 100,000 men in 1991.

Until recently, death rates, too, were edging steadily upward. In 1932, prostate cancer killed 17 of every 100,000 American men. By 1991, this number reached 25 of every 100,000. The figures for African-American men are even higher-55 of every 100,000. However, in the past several years, death rates, like incidence rates, appear to have been declining.

No one knows why prostate death rates went up. It is possible that, as more older men were diagnosed with prostate cancer, the disease was sometimes listed as the cause of death even when a man died of something else.

The reasons for the more recent death-rate decrease are also unclear, but the decrease may reflect improved treatment.

Risk Factors for Prostate Cancer

A **risk factor** is something that increases a person's chances of getting cancer. Risk factors don't necessarily cause cancer. Rather, they are indicators, statistically associated with an increase in a person's chances for getting a particular disease.

One risk factor for prostate cancer is age. Simply growing older increases a man's risk for getting prostate cancer. More than 75 percent of prostate cancer cases are diagnosed in men ages 65 or older; just 7 percent of cases occur in men younger than age 60. The average age at diagnosis is 72.

Another risk factor is race. African-American men have the world's highest incidence of prostate cancer-a third higher than white Americans. By contrast, Asian immigrants to the United States have much lower rates.

Family history also may play a role. For instance, risk increases for men whose father or brothers have prostate cancer. The risk is more than 10 times higher for a man who has three relatives with the disease. Risk may also be increased to some extent for men whose female relatives have a high incidence of breast cancer.

Researchers increasingly are looking at hormonal and **hereditary** factors and at diet, environmental exposures, and other lifestyle changes in relation to prostate cancer. For example, in countries such as China and Japan where low-fat diets are the norm, few men are diagnosed with prostate cancer. However, the incidence of prostate cancer is considerably higher among men who move from these countries to the United States, and the higher incidence persists in their sons' generation.

Researchers also are looking at the role of **vasectomy** in prostate cancer. Vasectomy is a surgical procedure that prevents men from fathering children. Some studies have suggested that vasectomies increase the risk of prostate cancer, although other studies failed to find such a link.

Symptoms of Prostate Cancer

Prostate cancer can grow quietly for years, which means most men with the disease have no obvious symptoms. When symptoms finally appear, they often are similar to those caused by prostate enlargement: difficulty urinating; a weak stream; a frequent urge to urinate, especially during the night; painful or burning urination; blood in the urine.

When cancer grows through the prostate capsule, it invades nearby tissues. It also may spread to the **lymph nodes** of the **pelvis**, or it may spread throughout the body (**metastasize**) via the bloodstream or the **lymphatic system**. Because prostate cancer tends to metastasize to the bone, bone pain, particularly in the back, can be another symptom of prostate cancer.

Early Detection of Prostate Cancer

Some doctors recommend screening for prostate cancer. Screening, as distinct from **diagnosis**, looks for signs of disease in people who have no cancer symptoms.

Screening for prostate cancer is controversial, because it is not yet known if the process actually saves lives, and it is not always clear that benefits outweigh the risks of diagnostic tests and treatments.

The main screening tools for prostate cancer are the DRE and the PSA test.

The higher a man's PSA level, the more likely that cancer could be in the picture. During screenings in men ages 50 or older, 85 of every 100 men will have normal PSA levels (4 ng/ml or below). Among the remaining 15 men, only 3 will have biopsies that show cancer.

Neither PSA nor DRE accurately identifies all cancers. The PSA test does a better job than DRE, but it still misses about one-third of cancers that are **clinically localized** (appear not to have grown through the prostate capsule).

It should be noted, though, that in spite of possible inaccuracy, most **tumors** that are found through screening are indeed early cancers.

Still, it is troublesome that PSA and DRE can falsely suggest cancer where none exists. Most men with an elevated PSA (or an abnormal DRE) go on to have additional diagnostic tests. Yet the majority of these men do not have cancer and will suffer needless anxiety.

Some recent refinements designed to make PSA testing more accurate and more precise are under **clinical study**. For instance, PSA density relates a man's PSA level to the size of his prostate, which can be estimated through ultrasound. **PSA velocity** is based on changes in PSA levels over time; a sharp rise from a baseline level raises the suspicion of cancer.

PSA circulates in the blood in two forms: free or attached to a **protein molecule**. In the case of a benign enlargement, there is more free PSA, while cancer produces more of the attached form, although the reasons for this difference are not well understood.

As for DRE, this test is most accurate when performed by a doctor who is highly skilled in such a procedure. But the procedure does have problems, often missing many small cancers, especially cancers toward the front of the prostate gland or deep within it. The exam also is notoriously unpopular among men and even among some doctors. Many men say they find the test embarrassing and uncomfortable. Studies also suggest that some physicians are reluctant to do rectal exams.

Even with early detection, there is as yet no proof that finding and treating **asymptomatic** prostate cancers do more good than harm. The reason: Many prostate cancers found through screening are slow-growing and might never cause symptoms. So far, it has not been possible to distinguish these slow-growing tumors from tumors that are **aggressive** and deadly. What is known is that treatment can have serious side effects, some of which are permanent.

Some insight into the detection dilemma could be forthcoming from the NCI's **Prostate, Lung, Colorectal, and Ovarian (PLCO) Cancer Screening Trial**. Some 37,000 men ages 55 to 74 are being screened, and those positive on either PSA or DRE will receive a diagnostic follow-up.

The study will determine if these men are less likely to die of prostate cancer than a comparison group of men who have not been screened.

The trial will also assess how well PSA levels correspond to the presence and size of a tumor.

When completed, this study, along with similar PSA/DRE studies that are going on in Europe, should make it clear whether the possible benefit of screening outweighs the harm.

In the meantime, each man needs to consult with his doctor and come to his own decision.

Do You Want To Be Screened?

The theoretical advantage of finding cancers early, before they cause symptoms, is that early cancers are less likely to have spread and may be easier to treat. Like other advanced cancers, advanced-stage prostate cancer can be a terrible disease.

But the disadvantage of screening is that it often leads to unnecessary additional diagnostic procedures.

Two basic questions still have no definitive answers: How frequently do the screening procedures such as PSA and DRE identify cancer? How frequently will finding prostate cancer produce a net benefit?

Studies designed to answer these questions are under way, but results won't be available for years. Earlier studies suffer from a variety of shortcomings, and none has proven that screening for prostate cancer decreases the risk of dying from the disease.

Lacking clear-cut answers, different organizations propose different guidelines. For example:

The American Cancer Society (ACS) recommends that both the PSA blood test and DRE should be offered annually to men ages 50 or older with at least a 10-year life expectancy. ACS adds that all men who are offered the option of screening should be given complete information on the benefits and risks of the procedures. African-American men or men with a strong family history of prostate cancer may be offered screening earlier, at age 45, for example. A strong family history means that prostate cancer has been detected in two or more first degree relatives such as a father or brother.

The American Urological Association endorses the American Cancer Society's screening policy: Men who choose to undergo screening should begin at age 50. However, men in high risk groups may begin at age 45.

The United States Preventive Services Task Force, its Canadian counterpart, and the American College of Physicians take a different position from that of the American Urological Association and the American Cancer Society: They recommend against the use of the PSA test for routine screening.

As you can see, opinions vary widely. Few doctors would recommend screening to a man older than age 80 or to a man in poor health. But for most men there is no "right" answer. It is important for you to make your own decision, taking into consideration the advice of your doctor and the best, most up-to-date information you can gather.

Do you want to be screened for prostate cancer?

In coming to your decision, it's important to consider how you would respond to a diagnosis of cancer. Prostate cancer is usually a slow-growing type of disease, but there are some fast-growing prostate cancers as well. Doctors can't always be sure what type of prostate cancer growth is present in your particular case. If you find out that you have prostate cancer, would you be able and willing to undergo surgery or radiotherapy, which carry the risk of incontinence and sexual impotence?

If you answer "yes," screening is an option. If "no," screening for prostate cancer may not be for you.

Diagnosing and Evaluating Prostate Cancer
Biopsy

Like other cancers, prostate cancer can actually be diagnosed only by examining tissue under a microscope. Whenever cancer is suspected, the diagnosis must be confirmed by a biopsy.

If your symptoms, the DRE, or your PSA test suggest cancer, your doctor will refer you to a urologist for a biopsy. The biopsy is typically performed in the urologist's office. The urologist gets an image of the prostate through a transrectal ultrasound probe. Then, to obtain tissue samples, the doctor inserts thin biopsy needles into areas of the gland that feel or look suspicious. Bits of tissue are removed from each site through the hollow needles. Each snip causes a sharp sting.

The tissue samples are then turned over to a **pathologist**, a doctor who specializes in the study of the microscopic cell and tissue changes produced by disease.

When a biopsy is prompted by an elevated PSA, rather than an abnormal area in the prostate gland detected by a rectal exam, the urologist may take random samples from six or more prostate areas. In a so-called **pattern biopsy**, the tissue samples are obtained from carefully spaced sectors of the gland; this helps establish the size and extent of any cancer.

Most men who have biopsies following routine exams do not have cancer. About three-quarters of the biopsies triggered by an abnormal DRE, and more than four-fifths of those instigated by an elevated PSA, reveal no cancer.

You may want to talk with your physician about the biopsy results. If there is any doubt about the diagnosis, you can get a second opinion from another pathologist.

Biopsies can miss cancer, too, about one time out of five. If your doctor strongly suspects cancer on clinical grounds, but the biopsy was negative, he or she may recommend a second biopsy.

If a Biopsy Is Positive

A diagnosis of prostate cancer obviously presents a man with complex decisions. He needs to understand the ramifications of the various options available to him. There are several levels, or **stages**, of prostate cancer, all of which call for different approaches to treatment. Moreover, for some stages of prostate cancer, there are several types of treatment, and it is not always clear which one is best. In fact, because treatment can produce some serious and life-long side effects-and because prostate cancer may grow very slowly-treatment may not always be better than no treatment.

Preventing Prostate Cancer

Researchers are investigating the possibility that drugs might keep latent prostate cancers from developing into active cancers. In the NCI's

Prostate Cancer Prevention Trial (PCPT), 18,000 healthy men age 55 or older are taking either finasteride (currently used to shrink the prostate in BPH) or a **placebo** every day for 7 to 10 years. Smaller trials are testing a variety of other medications or chemicals for their ability to prevent prostate cancer.

Since prostate cancer is less common in populations with low-fat, high-fiber diets, scientists are also looking into the possibility of using diet to prevent prostate cancer from developing. There is still no evidence to show that switching to a healthy diet after years of eating high-fat foods will make a difference, but small studies are testing the effects of a low-fat, high-soy diet among men who have an increased risk of prostate cancer and men who have already been treated for prostate cancer. One study found less prostate cancer among men who eat lots of tomato-based foods, especially tomato sauce cooked with a little olive oil.

This information hopefully has answered many of your questions about prostate cancer. However, no information can take the place of talking directly with your doctor. If you don't fully understand what the doctor is saying, ask him or her to explain further.

Understanding Back Problems

The human spine (or backbone) is made up of small bones called vertebrae. The vertebrae are stacked on top of each other to form a column. Between each vertebra is a cushion known as a disc. The vertebrae are held together by ligaments, and muscles are attached to the vertebrae by bands of tissue called tendons.

Openings in each vertebra line up to form a long hollow canal. The spinal cord runs through this canal from the base of the brain. Nerves from the spinal cord branch out and leave the spine through the spaces between the vertebrae.

The lower part of the back holds most of the body's weight. Even a minor problem with the bones, muscles, ligaments, or tendons in this area can cause pain when a person stand, bends, or moves around. Less often, a problem with a disc can pinch or irritate a nerve from the spinal cord, causing pain that runs down the leg, below the knee called sciatica.

Low back symptoms can keep you from doing your normal daily activities or doing things that you enjoy.

If you have been bothered by your lower back, you are not alone. Eight out of ten adults will have a low back problem at some time in their life. And most will have more than one episode of acute low back problems. In between episodes, most people return to their normal activities with little or no symptoms.

Causes of Low Back Problems

Even with today's technology, the exact reason or cause of low back problems can be found in very few people. Most times, the symptoms are blamed on poor muscle tone in the back, muscle tension or spasm, back sprains, ligament or muscle tears, joint problems. Sometimes nerves from the spinal cord can be irritated by "slipped" discs causing buttock or leg pain. This may also cause numbness, tingling, or weakness in the legs.

People who are in poor physical condition or do work that includes heavy labor or long periods of sitting or standing are at greater risk for low back problems.

These people also get better more slowly. Emotional stress or long periods of inactivity may make back symptoms seem worse.

Low back problems are often painful. But the good news is that very few people turn out to have a major problem with the bones or joints or the back or a dangerous medical conditions.

Things To Do About Low Back Problems
Seeing a health care provider

Many people who develop mild low back discomfort may not need to see a health care provider right away. Often, within a few days, the symptoms go away without any treatment.

A visit to your health care provider is good idea if:

Your symptoms are severe.

The pain is keeping you from doing things that you do every day.

The problem does not go away within a few days.

Your health care provider will check to see if you have a medical illness causing your back problem (chances are you will not). Your health care provider can also help you get some relief from your symptoms.

Your health care provider will:

Ask about your symptoms and what they keep you from doing.

Ask about your medical history.

Give you a physical exam.

Talking about your symptoms

Your health care provider will want to know about your back problem. Here are some examples of the kinds of questions he or she may ask you.

When did your back symptoms start?

Which of your daily activities are you not able to do because of your back symptoms?

Is there anything you do that makes the symptoms better or worse?

Have you noticed any problem with your legs?

Around the time your symptoms began, did you have a fever or symptoms of pain or burning when urinating?

Talking about your medical history

Be sure to tell your health care provider about your general health and about illnesses you have had in the past. Here are some questions your health care provider may ask you about your medical history.

Have you had a problem with your back in the past? If so, when?
What medical illnesses have you had (for example, cancer, arthritis, or diseases of the immune system)?
Which medicines do you take regularly?
Have you ever used intravenous (IV) drugs?
Have you recently lost weight without trying?

You should also tell your health care provider about anything you may be doing for your symptoms: medicines your are taking, creams or ointments you are using, and other home remedies.

Having a physical exam

Your health care provider will examine your back. Even after a careful physical examination, it may not be possible for your health care provider to tell you the exact cause of your low back problem. But you most likely will find out that your symptoms are not being caused by a dangerous medical condition. Very few people (about 1 in 200) have low back symptoms caused by such conditions. You probably won't need special tests if you have had low back symptoms for only a few weeks.

Getting Relief

Your health care provider will help you get relief from your pain, discomfort, or other symptoms. A number of medicines and other treatments help with low back symptoms. The good news is that most people start feeling better soon.

Proven treatments

Medicine often helps relieve low back symptoms. The type of medicine that your health care provider recommends depends on your symptoms and how uncomfortable you are.

If your symptoms are mild to moderate, you may get the relief you need from an over-the-counter (non-prescription) medicine such as acetaminophen, aspirin, or ibuprofen. These medicines usually have fewer side effects than prescription medicines and are less expensive.

If your symptoms are severe, your health care provider may recommend a prescription medicine.

For most people, medicine works well to control pain and discomfort. But any medicine can have side effects. For example, some people cannot take aspirin or ibuprofen because it can cause stomach irritation and even ulcers. Many medicines prescribed for low back pain can make people feel drowsy. These medicines should not be taken if you need to drive or use heavy equipment. Talk to your health care provider about the benefits and risks of any medicine recommended. If you develop side effects (such as nausea, vomiting, rash, dizziness), stop taking the medicine, and tell your health care provider right away.

Your health care provider may recommend one or more of the following to be used alone or along with medicine to help relieve your symptoms.

Heat or cold applied to the back. Within the first 48 hours after your back symptoms start, you may want apply a cold pack (or a bag of ice) to the painful area for 5 to 10 minutes at a time, If your symptoms last longer than 48 hours, you may find that a heating pad or hot shower or bath helps relieve your symptoms.

Spinal manipulation. This treatment (using the hands to apply force to the back to "adjust" the spine) can be helpful for some people in the first month of low back symptoms. It should only be done by a professional with experience in manipulation. You should go back to your health care provider if your symptoms have not responded to spinal manipulation within 4 weeks.

Keep in mind that everyone is different. You will have to find what works best to relieve your own back symptoms.

Other treatments

A number of other treatments are sometimes used for low back symptoms. While these treatments may give relief for a short time, none have been found to speed recovery or keep acute back problems from returning. They may also be expensive. Such treatments include:

Traction.

TENS (transcutaneous electrical nerve stimulation).

Massage.

Biofeedback

Acupuncture.

Injections into the back.

Back corsets.

Ultrasound.

Physical activity

Your health care provider will want to know about the physical demands of your life (your job or daily activities). Until you feel better, your health care provider may need to recommend some changes in your activities. You will want to talk to your health care provider about your own personal situation. In general, when pain is severe, you should avoid:

Heavy lifting.
Lifting when twisting, bending forward, and reaching.
Sitting for long periods of time.
The most important goal is for you to return to your normal activities as soon as it is safe. Your health care provider and (if you work) your employer can help you decide how much you are able to do safely at work. Your schedule can be gradually increased as your back improves.

Bed Rest

If your symptoms are sever, your health care provider may recommend a short period of bed rest. However, bed rest should be limited to 2 or 3 days. Lying down for longer periods may weaken muscles and bones and actually slow your recovery. If you feel that you must lie down, be sure to get up every few hours and walk around-even if it hurts. Feeling a little discomfort as you return to normal activity is common and does not mean that you are hurting yourself.

Back problems take time to get better. If your job or your normal daily activities make your back pain worse, it is important to communicate this to your family, supervisor, and coworkers. Put your energy into doing those things at work and at home that you are able to do comfortably. Be productive, but be clear about those tasks that you are not able to do.

Things You Can Do Now

While waiting for your back to improve, you may be able to make yourself more comfortable if you:
Wear comfortable, low-heeled shoes.
Make sure your work surface is at a comfortable height for you.
Use a chair with a good lower back support that may recline slightly.
If you must sit for long periods of time, try resting your feet on the floor or on a low stool, whichever is more comfortable.
If you must stand for long periods of time, try resting one foot on a low stool.
If you must drive long distances, try using a pillow or rolled-up towel behind the small of your back. Also, be sure to stop often and walk around for a few minutes.
If you have trouble sleeping, try sleeping on your back with a pillow under your knees, or sleep on your side with your knees bent and a pillow between your knees.

Exercise

A gradual return to normal activities, including exercise, is recommended. Exercise is important to your overall health and can help you to lose body fat (if needed). Even if you have mild to moderate low back symptoms, the following things can be done without putting much stress on your back:

Walking short distances.

Using a stationary bicycle.

Swimming.

It is important to start any exercise program slowly and to gradually build up the speed and length of time that your do the exercise. At first, you may find that your symptoms get a little worse when you exercise or become more active. Usually, this is nothing to worry about. However, if you pain becomes severe, contact your health care provider. Once you are able to return to normal activities comfortably, your health care provider may recommended further aerobic and back exercises.

If You Are Not Getting Better

Most low back problems get better quickly, and usually within 4 weeks. If your symptoms are not getting better within this time period, you should contact your health care provider.

Special tests

Your health care provider will examine your back again and may talk to you about getting some special tests. These may include x-rays, blood tests, or other special studies such as an MRI (magnetic resonance imaging) or CT (computerized tomography) scan of your back. These tests may help your health provider understand why you are not getting better. Your health care provider may also want to refer you to a specialist.

Certain things, such as stress (extra pressure at home or work), personal or emotional problems, depression, or a problem with drug or alcohol use can slow recovery or make back symptoms seem worse. If you have any of these problems, tell your health care provider.

Even having a lot of back pain does not by itself mean you need surgery. Surgery has been found to be helpful in only 1 in 100 cases of low back problems. In some people, surgery can even cause more problems. This is especially true if your only symptom is back pain.

People with certain nerve problems or conditions such as fractures or dislocations have the best chance of being helped by surgery. In most cases, however, decisions about surgery do not have to be made right away. Most back surgery can wait for several weeks without making the condition worse.

If your health care provider recommends surgery, be sure to ask about the reason for the surgery and about the risks and benefits you might expect. You may also want to get a second opinion.

Prevention of Low Back Problems

The best way to prevent low back problems is to stay fit. If you must lift something, even after your back seems better, be sure to:

Keep all lifted objects close to your body.

Avoid lifting while twisting, bending forward, and reaching.

You should continue to exercise even after your back symptoms have gone away. There are many exercises that can be done to condition muscles of your body and back. You should talk to your health care provider about the exercises that would be best for you.

When Low Back Symptoms Return

More than half of the people who recover from a first episode of acute low back symptoms will have another episode within a few years. Unless your back symptoms are very different from the first episode, or you have a new medical condition, you can expect to recover quickly and fully from each episode.

While Your Back is Getting Better

It is important to remember that even though you are having a problem with your back now, most likely it will begin to feel better soon. It is important to keep in mind that you are the most important person in taking care of your back and in helping to get back to your regular activities.

It may also help you to remember that:

Most low back problems last for a short amount of time and the symptoms usually get better with little or no medical treatment.

Low back problems can be painful. But pain rarely means that there is serious damage to your back.

Exercise can help you to feel better faster and prevent more back problems. A regular exercise program adds to your general health and may help you get back to the things you enjoy doing.

Understanding Breast Cancer

Breast cancer is hard to ignore. It is the most common form of cancer among American women, and almost everyone knows at least one person who has been treated for it.

Understandably, women are concerned about getting breast cancer, and this concern prompts them to watch for breast changes. Breast changes are common. Even though most are not cancer, they can be worrisome.

This information is designed to help you with these concerns. It describes screening for the early detection of breast cancer, explains the various types of breast changes that women experience, and outlines methods that doctors use to distinguish between benign (noncancerous) changes and cancer. It reviews factors that can increase a woman's cancer risk and reports on current approaches to breast cancer prevention.

This year in the United States an estimated 180,000 women will learn they have breast cancer. Three-fourths of the cases of breast cancer occur in women ages 50 or older, but it affects younger women, too (and about 1,400 men a year).

More women are getting breast cancer, but no one yet knows all the reasons why. Some of the increase can be traced to better ways of recognizing **cancer** and detecting cancers in an early stage. The increase also may be the result of changes in the way we live—postponing childbirth, taking replacement **hormones** and oral contraceptives, eating high-fat foods, or drinking more alcohol.

The encouraging news is that, more and more, breast cancer is being detected early, while the **tumor** is limited to the breast and very small. Currently, two-thirds of newly diagnosed breast cancers show no signs that the cancer has spread beyond the breast.

With prompt and appropriate treatment, the outlook for women with breast cancer is good. Moreover, a majority of women diagnosed with early stage breast cancer are candidates for treatment that saves the breast.

The key to finding breast cancer is early detection, and the key to early detection is screening: looking for cancer in women who have no symptoms of disease. The best available tool is a regular **screening mammogram—x-ray** of the breast—coupled with a **clinical breast exam**—by a doctor or nurse.

Mammography A **mammogram** is an x-ray of the breast. Cancers that are found on mammograms but that cannot be felt (**nonpalpable cancers**) usually are smaller than cancers that can be felt, and they are less likely to have spread.

Two Kinds of Mammography: Diagnostic and Screening
If a woman visits her doctor because of unusual breast changes such as a lump, pain, nipple thickening or discharge, or changes in breast size or shape, or has a suspicious screening mammogram, the doctor often asks her to have a **diagnostic mammogram**: an x-ray of the breast to help assess her symptoms. A diagnostic mammogram is a basic medical tool, and it is appropriate for women of any age.
What Are the Benefits of Screening Mammography?
High-quality mammography is the most effective tool now available to detect breast cancer early, before symptoms appear—often before a breast lump can even be felt. Regularly scheduled mammograms can decrease a woman's chance of dying from breast cancer. For some women, early detection may prevent the need to remove the entire breast or receive chemotherapy.
Who Benefits From Screening Mammography?

Studies done over the past 30 years clearly show that regular screening mammography significantly reduces the death rate from breast cancer in women over the age of 50. Recent results from studies show that regular mammography also reduces death rates from breast cancer in women who begin screening in their forties.
The effectiveness of mammography seems to increase as a woman ages, and the time it takes for benefits to emerge appears to take longer in younger women.
Who Is at Average Risk for Breast Cancer?
Simply being a woman and getting older puts you at average **risk** for developing breast cancer. The older you are, the greater your chance of getting breast cancer. No woman should consider herself too old to need regular screening mammograms.
Who Is at Higher Than Average Risk for Breast Cancer?
One or more of the following conditions place a woman at higher than average risk for breast cancer:
personal history of a prior breast cancer

mother, sister, daughter, or two or more close relatives, such as cousins, with a history of breast cancer (especially if diagnosed at a young age)

a diagnosis of a breast condition that may predispose a woman to breast cancer (i.e., **atypical hyperplasia**), or a history of two or more breast biopsies for benign breast disease.

Also playing a role in a heightened risk for breast cancer is **breast density.** Women ages 45 or older who have at least 75 percent dense tissue on a mammogram are at elevated risk. And a slight increase in the risk of breast cancer is associated with having a first birth at age 30 or older.

In addition, women who receive chest irradiation for conditions such as Hodgkin's disease at age 30 or younger remain at higher risk for breast cancer throughout their lives. These women require meticulous surveillance for breast cancer.

These factors that increase cancer risk—**risk factors**—do not by themselves cause cancer. Having one or more does not mean that you are certain or even likely to develop breast cancer. Even among women with no other risk factors except a strong family history—for example, both a mother and a sister or two sisters with early onset breast cancer—three-fourths will not develop the disease.

What Are the Limitations of Screening Mammography?

Early detection by mammography does not guarantee that a woman's life will be saved. It may not help a woman who has a fast-growing cancer that has spread to other parts of her body before being detected. Also, about half of the women whose breast cancers are detected by mammography would not have died from cancer, even if they had waited until the lump could be felt, because their tumors are slow-growing and treatable.

False Negative Mammograms

Breasts of younger women contain many glands and ligaments. Because their breasts appear dense on mammograms, it is difficult to see tumors or to distinguish between normal and abnormal breast conditions. As a woman grows older, the glandular and fibrous tissues of her breasts gradually give way to less dense fatty tissues. Mammograms can then see into the breast tissue more easily to detect abnormal changes. About 25 percent of breast tumors are missed in women in their forties, compared to about 10 percent of women older than age 50. These are called **false negatives**. A normal mammogram in a woman with symptoms does not rule out breast cancer. Sometimes a clinical breast exam by a doctor or nurse can reveal a breast lump that is missed by a mammogram.

False Positive Mammograms

Between 5 and 10 percent of mammogram results are abnormal and require more testing (more mammograms, fine needle **aspiration**, **ultrasound**, or **biopsy**), and most of the follow-up tests confirm that no cancer was present. It is estimated that a woman who has yearly mammograms between ages 40 and 49 would have about a 30 percent chance of having a **false positive** mammogram at some point in that decade, and about a 7 to 8 percent chance of having a breast biopsy within the 10-year period. The estimate for false positive mammograms is about 25 percent for women ages 50 or older.

Increased Cases of Ductal Carcinoma In Situ (DCIS)

The increased use of screening mammography has increased the detection of small abnormal tissue growths confined to the milk ducts in the breast, called **ductal carcinoma in situ (DCIS)**. Doctors don't know which, if any, cases of DCIS may become life threatening. Usually, the growth is removed surgically, and **radiation** treatment is often given.

How Mammograms Are Made Mammography is a simple procedure. It uses a "dedicated" x-ray machine specifically designed for x-raying the breast and used only for that purpose (in contrast to machines used to take x-rays of the bones or other parts of the body). The standard screening exam includes two views of each breast, one from above and one angled from the side. A registered technologist places the breast between two flat plastic plates. The two plates are then pressed together. The idea is to flatten the breast as much as possible; spreading the tissue out makes any abnormal details easier to spot with a minimum of radiation. The technologist takes the x-ray, then repeats the procedure for the next view.

The pressure from the plates may be uncomfortable, or even somewhat painful. It helps to remember that each x-ray takes less than one minute—and it could save your life. It also helps to schedule mammography just after your period, when your breasts are least likely to be tender, or at the same time each year, if you no longer have your period.

Although some women are concerned about radiation exposure, the risk of any harm is extremely small. The doses of radiation used for mammography are very low and considered safe. The exact amount of radiation needed for a specific mammogram will depend on several factors. For instance, breasts that are large or dense will require higher doses to get a clear image. Federal mammography guidelines limit the radiation used for each exposure of the breast to 0.3 **rad**. (A "rad" is a unit of measurement that stands for **r**adiation **a**bsorbed **d**ose.) In practice, most mammograms deliver just a small fraction of this amount.

Specialized mammography facilities have experienced personnel as well as modern equipment that is custom designed for mammograms. The combination of good technology and expertise makes it possible to obtain good-quality x-ray images with very low doses of radiation.

Reading a Mammogram The mammogram is first checked by the technologist and then read by a diagnostic **radiologist**, a doctor who specializes in interpreting x-rays. The radiologist looks for unusual shadows, masses, distortions, special patterns of tissue density, and differences between the two breasts. The shape of a mass can be important, too. A growth that is **benign** (noncancerous) such as a cyst, looks smooth and round and has a clearly defined edge. Breast cancer, in contrast, often has an irregular outline with finger-like extensions.

Many mammograms show nontransparent white specks. These are calcium deposits known as calcifications.

Macrocalcifications are usually associated with benign breast conditions; many clusters of macrocalcifications in one area may be an early sign of breast cancer.

The radiologist will report the findings from your mammogram directly to you or to your doctor, who will contact you with the results. If you need further tests or exams, your doctor will let you know. If you don't get a report, you should call and ask for the results.

Your mammograms are an important part of your health history. Being able to compare earlier mammograms with new ones helps your doctor evaluate areas that look suspicious. If you move, ask your radiologist for your films and hand-carry them to your new physician, so they can be kept with your file. Always make sure that the radiologist who reads your mammogram has the old films to use for comparison.

Mammograms and Breast Implants A woman who has had **breast implants** should continue to have mammograms. (A woman who has had an implant following breast cancer surgery should ask her doctor whether a mammogram is still necessary.) However, the woman should inform the technologist and radiologist beforehand and make sure they are experienced in x-raying patients with breast implants.

Because silicone implants are not transparent on x-ray, they can block a clear view of the tissues behind them. This is especially true if the implant has been placed in front of, rather than beneath, the chest muscles.

Experienced technologists and radiologists know how to carefully compress the breasts to avoid rupturing the implant. They can also use special techniques to detect abnormalities, sliding the implant backward against the chest wall, and pulling the breast tissue over and in front of it. Interpreting the mammogram can also be difficult, especially if scar tissue has formed around the implant or if silicone has leaked into nearby breast tissues.

Choose a Mammography Facility Many places—breast clinics, radiology departments of hospitals, mobile vans, private radiology practices, doctors' offices—offer high-quality mammography. Your doctor can arrange for a mammogram for you, or you can schedule the appointment yourself.

In addition to quality, another important consideration is cost. Most screening mammograms cost between $50 and $150. Most states now have laws requiring health insurance companies to reimburse all or part of the cost of screening mammograms; check with your insurance company. Medicare pays some of the cost for screening mammograms; check with your health care provider.

Some health service agencies and some employers provide mammograms free or at low cost. Low cost does not mean low quality, however. A large government survey found that some of the facilities charging the lowest fees (often because they serve large numbers of women) were among the best in terms of complying with high-quality standards.

Schedule a Regular Mammogram Early detection of breast cancer is crucial for successful treatment, and regular screening mammography is currently the best tool for early detection. A survey by the National Center for Health Statistics found that 60 percent of all women ages 40 to 49 got a mammogram in the preceding 2 years, and 65 percent of women ages 50 to 64 had done so, but only 54 percent of women ages 65 and over had been screened during that time. It is clear that many women still do not get mammograms at regular intervals. Sadly, the women least likely to have regular exams include those at highest risk, women ages 60 and older.

The reason women most frequently give for having—or not having—a mammogram is whether or not the doctor suggested it. Although surveys show that more doctors routinely advise women about mammography, some fail to do so—because they forget, or because they assume that another doctor has done so. If your doctor doesn't suggest mammography, it will be up to you to raise the issue.

Other Techniques for Detecting Breast Cancer

Clinical Breast Exam

Most professional medical organizations recommend that a woman have periodic breast exams by a doctor or nurse along with getting regular screening mammograms. You may find it convenient to schedule a breast exam during your routine physical.

The examiner will look at your breasts while you are sitting and while you are lying down. You may be asked to raise your arms over your head or let them hang by your sides, or to press your hands against your hips. The examiner checks your breasts carefully for changes in the skin such as dimpling, scaling, or puckering; any discharge from the nipples; or any difference in appearance between the two breasts, including differences in size or shape. The next step is **palpation**: Using the pads of the fingers to feel for lumps, the examiner will systematically inspect the entire breast, the underarm, and the collarbone area, first on one side, then on the other.

A lump is generally the size of a pea before a skilled examiner can detect it. Lumps that are soft, round, and smooth tend not to be cancerous. An irregular, hard lump that feels firmly anchored within the breast tissue is more likely to be a cancer. However, these are general observations, not hard and fast rules.

A breast exam by a doctor or nurse can find some cancers missed by mammography, even very small ones. In addition to the skill and carefulness of the examiner, the success of a physical exam can be influenced by your monthly cycle and by the size of your breast, as well as by the size and location of the lump itself. Lumps are harder to find in a large breast.

Currently, mammography and breast exams by the doctor or nurse are the most common and useful techniques for finding breast cancer early. Other methods such as ultrasound may be helpful in clarifying the diagnosis for women who have suspicious breast changes. However, no other procedure has yet proven to be more effective than mammography for screening women with no symptoms; thus, most alternative methods of breast cancer detection are used primarily in medical research programs.

Ultrasound

Ultrasound works by sending high-frequency sound waves into the breast. The pattern of echoes from these sound waves is converted into an image (**sonogram**) of the breast's interior. Ultrasound, which is painless and harmless, can distinguish between tumors that are solid and cysts, which are filled with fluid. Sonograms of the breast can also help radiologists to evaluate some lumps that can be felt but are hard to see on a mammogram, especially in the dense breasts of young women. Unlike mammography, ultrasound cannot detect the microcalcifications that sometimes indicate cancer, nor does it pick up small tumors.

CT Scanning

Computed tomography, or **CT scanning**, uses a computer to organize and stack the information from multiple x-ray, cross-sectional views of a body's organ or area. The scans are made by having the source of an x-ray beam rotate around the patient. X-rays passing through the body are detected by sensors that pass the information to computers. Once processed, the information is displayed as an image on a video screen. CT can separate overlapping structures precisely and is sometimes helpful in locating breast abnormalities that are difficult to pinpoint with mammography or ultrasound—for instance, a tumor that is so close to the chest wall that it shows up in only one mammographic view.

Research on New Techniques

Several new techniques for imaging the breast are in the research stage. These include the use of **magnetic resonance imaging (MRI)** and **positron emission tomography (PET scanning)** to identify tissues that are abnormally active. MRI uses a large magnet to surround the patient along with radio frequencies and a computer to produce its images. PET scanning uses signals from radioactive traces to construct images. **Laser beam scanning** shines a powerful laser beam through the breast, while a special camera on the far side of the breast records the image.

Researchers are also striving to improve the detection power and diagnostic accuracy of mammography. **Digital mammography** is a technique for recording x-ray images in computer code, improving the detection of breast abnormalities. **Computer-aided diagnosis**, or **CAD**, uses special computer programs to scan mammographic images and alert radiologists to areas that look suspicious.

Over her lifetime, a woman can encounter a broad variety of breast conditions. These include normal changes that occur during the **menstrual cycle** as well as several types of benign lumps. What they have in common is that they are not cancer. Even for breast lumps that require a biopsy, some 80 percent prove to be benign.

Each breast has 15 to 20 sections, called **lobes**, each with many smaller **lobules**. The lobules end in dozens of tiny **bulbs** that can produce milk. Lobes, lobules, and bulbs are all linked by thin tubes called **ducts**. These ducts lead to the nipple, which is centered in a dark area of skin called the **areola**. The spaces between the lobules and ducts are filled with fat. There are no muscles in the breast, but muscles lie under each breast and cover the ribs.

These normal features can sometimes make the breasts feel lumpy, especially in women who are thin or who have small breasts.

In addition, from the time a girl begins to menstruate, her breasts undergo regular changes each month. Many doctors believe that nearly all breasts develop some lasting changes, beginning when the woman is about 30 years old. Eventually, about half of all women will experience symptoms such as lumps, pain, or **nipple discharge**. Generally these disappear with menopause.

Some studies show that the chances of developing **benign breast changes** are higher for a woman who has never had children, has irregular menstrual cycles, or has a family history of breast cancer. Benign breast conditions are less common among women who take birth control pills or who are overweight. Because they generally involve the glandular tissues of the breast, benign breast conditions are more of a problem for women of child-bearing age, who have more glandular breasts.

Types of Benign Breast Changes Common benign breast changes fall into several broad categories. These include generalized breast changes, solitary lumps, nipple discharge, and **infection** and/or **inflammation**.

Generalized Breast Changes

Generalized breast lumpiness is known by several names, including **fibrocystic disease** changes and benign breast disease. Such lumpiness, which is sometimes described as "ropy" or "granular," can often be felt in the area around the nipple and areola and in the upper-outer part of the breast. Such lumpiness may become more obvious as a woman approaches middle age and the milk-producing glandular tissue of her breasts increasingly gives way to soft, fatty tissue. Unless she is taking replacement hormones, this type of lumpiness generally disappears for good after **menopause**.

The menstrual cycle also brings **cyclic breast changes**. Many women experience swelling, tenderness, and pain before and sometimes during their periods. At the same time, one or more lumps or a feeling of increased lumpiness may develop because of extra fluid collecting in the breast tissue. These lumps normally go away by the end of the period.

During pregnancy, the milk-producing glands become swollen and the breasts may feel lumpier than usual. Although very uncommon, breast cancer has been diagnosed during pregnancy. If you have any questions about how your breasts feel or look, talk to your doctor.

Solitary Lumps

Benign breast conditions also include several types of distinct, solitary lumps. Such lumps, which can appear at any time, may be large or small, soft or rubbery, fluid-filled or solid.

Cysts are fluid-filled sacs. They occur most often in women ages 35 to 50, and they often enlarge and become tender and painful just before the menstrual period. They are usually found in both breasts. Some cysts are so small they cannot be felt; rarely, cysts may be several inches across. Cysts are usually treated by observation or by fine needle aspiration.

Fibroadenomas are solid and round benign tumors that are made up of both structural (fibro) and glandular (adenoma) tissues. Usually, these lumps are painless and found by the woman herself. They feel rubbery and can easily be moved around. Fibroadenomas are the most common type of tumors in women in their late teens and early twenties, and they occur twice as often in African-American women as in other American women.

Fibroadenomas have a typically benign appearance on mammography (smooth, round masses with a clearly defined edge), and they can sometimes be diagnosed with fine needle aspiration. Although fibroadenomas do not become malignant, they can enlarge with pregnancy and breast-feeding. Most surgeons believe that it is a good idea to remove fibroadenomas to make sure they are benign.

Fat necrosis is the name given to painless, round, and firm lumps formed by damaged and disintegrating fatty tissues. This condition typically occurs in obese women with very large breasts. It often develops in response to a bruise or blow to the breast, even though the woman may not remember the specific injury. Sometimes the skin around the lumps looks red or bruised. Fat necrosis can easily be mistaken for cancer, so such lumps are removed in a surgical biopsy.

Sclerosing adenosis is a benign condition involving the excessive growth of tissues in the breast's lobules. It frequently causes breast pain. Usually the changes are microscopic, but adenosis can produce lumps, and it can show up on a mammogram, often as calcifications. Short of biopsy, adenosis can be difficult to distinguish from cancer. The usual approach is surgical biopsy, which furnishes both diagnosis and treatment.

Nipple Discharge

Nipple discharge accompanies some benign breast conditions. Since the breast is a gland, secretions from the nipple of a mature woman are not unusual, nor even necessarily a sign of disease. For example, small amounts of discharge commonly occur in women taking birth control pills or certain other medications, including sedatives and tranquilizers. If the discharge is being caused by a disease, the disease is more likely to be benign than cancerous.

Nipple discharges come in a variety of colors and textures. A milky discharge can be traced to many causes, including thyroid malfunction and oral contraceptives or other drugs. Women with generalized breast lumpiness may have a sticky discharge that is brown or green.

The doctor will take a sample of the discharge and send it to a laboratory to be analyzed. Benign sticky discharges are treated chiefly by keeping the nipple clean. A discharge caused by infection may require antibiotics.

One of the most common sources of a bloody or sticky discharge is an **intraductal papilloma**, a small, wartlike growth that projects into breast ducts near the nipple. Any slight bump or bruise in the area of the nipple can cause the papilloma to bleed. Single (solitary) intraductal papillomas usually affect women nearing menopause. If the discharge becomes bothersome, the diseased duct can be removed surgically without damaging the appearance of the breast. Multiple intraductal papillomas, in contrast, are more common in younger women. They often occur in both breasts and are more likely to be associated with a lump than with nipple discharge. Multiple intraductal papillomas, or any papillomas associated with a lump, need to be removed.

Infection and/or Inflammation

Infection and/or inflammation, including **mastitis** and **mammary duct ectasia**, are characteristic of some benign breast conditions.

Mastitis (sometimes called "postpartum mastitis") is an infection most often seen in women who are breast-feeding. A duct may become blocked, allowing milk to pool, causing inflammation, and setting the stage for infection by bacteria. The breast appears red and feels warm, tender, and lumpy.

In its earlier stages, mastitis can be cured by antibiotics. If a pus-containing **abscess** forms, it will need to be drained or surgically removed.

Mammary duct ectasia is a disease of women nearing menopause. Ducts beneath the nipple become inflamed and can become clogged. Mammary duct ectasia can become painful, and it can produce a thick and sticky discharge that is grey to green in color. Treatment consists of warm compresses, antibiotics, and, if necessary, surgery to remove the duct.

Benign Breast Conditions and the Risk for Breast Cancer Most benign breast changes do not increase a woman's risk for getting cancer. Recent studies show that only certain very specific types of microscopic changes put a woman at higher risk. These changes feature excessive cell growth, or **hyperplasia**.

About 70 percent of the women who have a biopsy showing a benign condition have *no* evidence of hyperplasia. **These women are at no increased risk for breast cancer.**

About 25 percent of benign breast biopsies show signs of hyperplasia, including conditions such as intraductal papilloma and sclerosing adenosis. Hyperplasia *slightly* increases the risk of developing breast cancer.

The remaining 5 percent of benign breast biopsies reveal both excessive cell growth—hyperplasia—and cells that are abnormal—atypia. A diagnosis of atypical hyperplasia, as it is called, *moderately* increases breast cancer risk.

If You Find a Lump If you discover a lump in one breast, check the other breast. If both breasts feel the same, the lumpiness is probably normal. You should, however, mention it to your doctor at your next visit.

But if the lump is something new or unusual and does not go away after your next menstrual period, it is time to call your doctor. The same is true if you discover a discharge from the nipple or skin changes such as dimpling or puckering. If you do not have a doctor, your local medical society may be able to help you find one in your area.

You should not let fear delay you. It is natural to be concerned if you find a lump in your breast. But remember that four-fifths of all breast lumps are not cancer. The sooner any problem is diagnosed, the sooner you can have it treated.

Clinical Evaluation

No matter how your breast lump was discovered, the doctor will want to begin with your medical history. What symptoms do you have and how long have you had them? What is your age, menstrual status, general health? Are you pregnant? Are you taking any medications? How many children do you have? Do you have any relatives with benign breast conditions or breast cancer? Have you previously been diagnosed with benign breast changes?

The doctor will then carefully examine your breasts and will probably schedule you for a diagnostic mammogram, to obtain as much information as possible about the changes in your breast. This may be either a lump that can be felt or an abnormality discovered on a screening mammogram. Diagnostic mammography may include additional views or use special techniques to magnify a suspicious area or to eliminate shadows produced by overlapping layers of normal breast tissue. The doctor will want to compare the diagnostic mammograms with any previous mammograms. If the lump appears to be a cyst, your doctor may ask you to have a sonogram (ultrasound study).

Aspirating a Cyst

When a cyst is suspected, some doctors proceed directly with aspiration. This procedure, which uses a very thin needle and a syringe, takes only a few minutes and can be done in the doctor's office. The procedure is not usually very uncomfortable, since most of the nerves in the breast are in the skin.

Holding the lump steady, the doctor inserts the needle and attempts to draw out any fluid. If the lump is indeed a cyst, removing the fluid will cause the cyst to collapse and the lump to disappear. Unless the cyst reappears in the next week or two, no other treatment is needed. If the cyst reappears at a later date, it can simply be drained again.

If the lump turns out to be solid, it may be possible to use the needle to withdraw a clump of cells, which can then be sent to a laboratory for further testing. (Cysts are so rarely associated with cancer that the fluid removed from a cyst is not usually tested unless it is bloody or the woman is older than 55 years of age.)

Biopsy The only certain way to learn whether a breast lump or mammographic abnormality is cancerous is by having a biopsy, a procedure in which tissue is removed by a surgeon or other specialist and examined under a microscope by a **pathologist**. A pathologist is a doctor who specializes in identifying tissue changes that are characteristic of disease, including cancer.

Tissue samples for biopsy can be obtained by either surgery or needle. The doctor's choice of biopsy technique depends on such things as the nature and location of the lump, as well as the woman's general health.

Surgical biopsies can be either excisional or incisional. An **excisional biopsy** removes the entire lump or suspicious area. Excisional biopsy is currently the standard procedure for lumps that are smaller than an inch or so in diameter. In effect, it is similar to a **lumpectomy**, surgery to remove the lump and a margin of surrounding tissue. Lumpectomy is usually used in combination with radiation therapy as the basic treatment for early breast cancer.

An excisional biopsy is typically performed in the outpatient department of a hospital. A local anesthetic is injected into the woman's breast. Sometimes she is given a tranquilizer before the procedure. The surgeon makes an incision along the contour of the breast and removes the lump along with a small margin of normal tissue. Because no skin is removed, the biopsy scar is usually small. The procedure typically takes less than an hour. After spending an hour or two in the recovery room, the woman goes home the same day.

An **incisional biopsy** removes only a portion of the tumor (by slicing into it) for the pathologist to examine. Incisional biopsies are generally reserved for tumors that are larger. They too are usually performed under local anesthesia, with the woman going home the same day.

Whether or not a surgical biopsy will change the shape of your breast depends partly on the size of the lump and where it is located in the breast, as well as how much of a margin of healthy tissue the surgeon decides to remove. You should talk with your doctor beforehand, so you understand just how extensive the surgery will be and what the cosmetic result will be.

Needle biopsies can be performed with either a very fine needle or a cutting needle large enough to remove a small nugget of tissue.

Fine needle aspiration uses a very thin needle and syringe to remove either fluid from a cyst or clusters of cells from a solid mass. Accurate fine needle aspiration biopsy of a solid mass takes great skill, gained through experience with numerous cases.

Core needle biopsy uses a somewhat larger needle with a special cutting edge. The needle is inserted, under local anesthesia, through a small incision in the skin, and a small core of tissue is removed. This technique may not work well for lumps that are very hard or very small. Core needle biopsy may cause some bruising, but rarely leaves an external scar, and the procedure is over in a matter of minutes.

At some institutions with extensive experience, aspiration biopsy is considered as reliable as surgical biopsy; it is trusted to confirm the **malignancy** of a clinically suspicious mass or to confirm a diagnosis that a lump is not cancerous. Should the needle biopsy results be uncertain, the diagnosis is pursued with a surgical biopsy. Some doctors prefer to verify all aspiration biopsy results with a surgical biopsy before proceeding with treatment.

Localization biopsy (also known as needle localization) is a procedure that uses mammography to locate and a needle to biopsy breast abnormalities that can be seen on a mammogram but cannot be felt (nonpalpable abnormalities). Localization can be used with surgical biopsy, fine needle aspiration, or core needle biopsy.

For a surgical biopsy, the radiologist locates the abnormality on a mammogram (or a sonogram) just prior to surgery. Using the mammogram as a guide, the radiologist inserts a fine needle or wire so the tip rests in the suspicious area—typically, an area of microcalcifications. The needle is anchored with a gauze bandage, and a second mammogram is taken to confirm that the needle is on target.

The woman, along with her mammograms, goes to the operating room, where the surgeon locates and cuts out the needle-targeted area. The more precisely the needle is placed, the less tissue needs to be removed.

Sometimes the surgeon will be able to feel the lump during surgery. In other cases, especially where the mammogram showed only microcalcifications, the abnormality can be neither seen nor felt. To make sure the surgical specimen in fact contains the abnormality, it is x-rayed on the spot. If this **specimen x-ray** fails to show the mass or the calcifications, the surgeon is able to remove additional tissue.

Stereotactic localization biopsy is a newer approach that relies on a three-dimensional x-ray to guide the needle biopsy of a nonpalpable mass. With one type of equipment, the patient lies face down on an examining table with a hole in it that allows the breast to hang through; the x-ray machine and the maneuverable needle "gun" are set up underneath. Alternatively, specialized stereotactic equipment can be attached to a standard mammography machine.

The breast is x-rayed from two different angles, and a computer plots the exact position of the suspicious area. (Because only a small area of the breast is exposed to the radiation, the doses are similar to those from standard mammography.) Once the target is clearly identified, the radiologist positions the gun and advances the biopsy needle into the lesion.

Tissue Studies

The cells or tissue removed through needle or surgical biopsy are promptly sent (along with the x-ray of the specimen, if one was made) to the pathology lab. If the excised lump is large enough, the pathologist can take a preliminary look by quick-freezing a small portion of the tissue sample. This makes the sample firm enough to slice into razor-thin sections that can be examined under the microscope. A "**frozen section**" provides an immediate, if provisional, diagnosis, and the surgeon may be able to give you the results before you go home.

The results of a frozen section are not 100 percent certain, however. A more thorough assessment takes several days, while the pathologist processes "**permanent sections**" of tissue that can be examined in greater detail.

When the biopsy specimen is small—as is often the case when the abnormality consists of mammographic calcifications only—many doctors prefer to bypass a frozen section so the tiny specimen can be analyzed in its entirety.

The pathologist looks for abnormal cell shapes and unusual growth patterns. In many cases the diagnosis will be clear-cut. However, the distinctions between benign and cancerous can be subtle, and even experts don't always agree. When in doubt, pathologists readily consult their colleagues. If there is any question about the results of your biopsy, you will want to make sure your biopsy slides have been reviewed by more than one pathologist.

Deciding To Biopsy

Not every lump or mammographic change merits a biopsy. Nearly all mammographic masses that look smooth and clearly outlined, for instance, are benign. Your doctor needs to thoughtfully weigh the findings from your physical exam and mammogram along with your background and your medical history when making a recommendation about a biopsy.

Although benign lumps rarely, if ever, turn into cancer, cancerous lumps can develop near benign lumps and can be hidden on a mammogram. Even if you have had a benign lump removed in the past, you cannot be sure any new lump is also benign.

In some cases, the doctor may suggest watching the suspicious area for a month or two. Because many lumps are caused by normal hormonal changes, this waiting period may provide additional information.

Similarly, if the changes on your mammogram show all the signs of benign disease, your doctor may advise waiting several months and then taking another mammogram. This would be followed by more diagnostic mammograms over the next three years. If you choose this option, however, you must be strongly committed to regularly scheduled follow-ups.

If you feel uncomfortable about waiting, express your concerns to your doctor. You may also want to get a second opinion, perhaps from a breast specialist or surgeon. Many cities have breast clinics where you can get a second opinion.

Biopsy: One Step or Two?

Not too many years ago, all women undergoing surgery for breast symptoms had a **one-step procedure**: If the surgical biopsy showed cancer, the surgeon performed a **mastectomy** immediately. The woman went into surgery not knowing if she had cancer or if her breast would be removed.

Today a woman facing biopsy has a broader range of options. In most cases, biopsy and diagnosis will be separated from any further treatment by an interval of several days or weeks. Such a **two-step procedure** does not harm the patient, and it has several benefits. It allows time for the tissue sample to be examined in detail and, if cancer is found, it gives the woman time to adjust to the diagnosis. She can review her treatment options, seek a second opinion, receive counseling, and arrange her schedule.

Some women, nonetheless, prefer a one-step procedure. They have decided beforehand that, if the surgical biopsy and frozen section show cancer, they want to go ahead with surgery, either mastectomy or lumpectomy and axillary dissection (removal of the underarm lymph nodes). If, on the other hand, the lump proves to be benign, the incision will be closed. The procedure will have taken less than an hour, and the woman may go home the same day or the next day.

A one-step procedure avoids the physical and psychological stress, as well as the costs in time and money, of two rounds of surgery and anesthesia—a particularly important consideration for women who are ill or frail. Women who have symptoms of breast cancer can find the wait between biopsy and surgery emotionally draining, and they may be relieved to have a one-step procedure to take care of the problem as quickly as possible.

No single solution is right for everyone. Each woman should consult with her doctors and her family, weigh the alternatives, and decide what approach is appropriate. Being involved in the decision-making process can give a woman a sense of control over her body and her life.

Arthritis Pain

What Is Arthritis?

The word arthritis literally means joint inflammation, but is often used to refer to a group of more than 100 rheumatic diseases that can cause pain, stiffness, and swelling in the joints. These diseases may affect not only the joints but also other parts of the body, including important supporting structures such as muscles, bones, tendons, and ligaments, as well as some internal organs. This fact sheet focuses on pain caused by two of the most common forms of arthritis—osteoarthritis and rheumatoid arthritis.

What Is Pain?

Pain is the body's warning system, alerting you that something is wrong. The International Association for the Study of Pain defines it as an unpleasant experience associated with actual or potential tissue damage to a person's body. Specialized nervous system cells (neurons) that transmit pain signals are found throughout the skin and other body tissues. These cells respond to things such as injury or tissue damage. For example, when a harmful agent such as a sharp knife comes in contact with your skin, chemical signals travel from neurons in the skin through nerves in the spinal cord to your brain, where they are interpreted as pain.

Most forms of arthritis are associated with pain that can be divided into two general categories: acute and chronic. Acute pain is temporary. It can last a few seconds or longer but wanes as healing occurs. Some examples of things that cause acute pain include burns, cuts, and fractures. Chronic pain, such as that seen in people with osteoarthritis and rheumatoid arthritis, ranges from mild to severe and can last a lifetime.

How Many Americans Suffer From Arthritis Pain?

Chronic pain is a major health problem in the United States and is one of the most weakening effects of arthritis. More than 40 million Americans suffer from some form of arthritis, and many have chronic pain that limits daily activity. Osteoarthritis is by far the most common form of arthritis, affecting about 20 million Americans, while rheumatoid arthritis, which affects about 2.1 million Americans, is the most crippling form of the disease.

What Causes Arthritis Pain? Why Is It So Variable?

The pain of arthritis may come from different sources. These may include inflammation of the synovial membrane (tissue that lines the joints), the tendons, or the ligaments; muscle strain; and fatigue. A combination of these factors contributes to the intensity of the pain.

The pain of arthritis varies greatly from person to person, for reasons that doctors do not yet understand completely. Factors that contribute to the pain include swelling within the joint, the amount of heat or redness present, or damage that has occurred within the joint. In addition, activities affect pain differently so that some patients note pain in their joints after first getting out of bed in the morning whereas others develop pain after prolonged use of the joint. Each individual has a different threshold and tolerance for pain, often affected by both physical and emotional factors. These can include depression, anxiety, and even hypersensitivity at the affected sites due to inflammation and tissue injury. This increased sensitivity appears to affect the amount of pain perceived by the individual. Social support networks can make an important contribution to pain management.

How Do Doctors Measure Arthritis Pain?

Pain is a private, unique experience that cannot be seen. The most common way to measure pain is for the doctor to ask you, the patient, about your difficulties. For example, the doctor may ask you to describe the level of pain you feel on a scale of 1 to 10. You may use words like aching, burning, stinging, or throbbing. These words will give the doctor a clearer picture of the pain you are experiencing.

Since doctors rely on your description of pain to help guide treatment, you may want to keep a pain diary to record your pain sensations. You can begin a week or two before your visit to the doctor. On a daily basis, you can describe the situations that cause or alter the intensity of your pain, the sensations and severity of your pain, and your reactions to the pain. For example: "On Monday night, sharp pains in my knees produced by housework interfered with my sleep; on Tuesday morning, because of the pain, I had a hard time getting out bed. However, I coped with the pain by taking my medication and applying ice to my knees." The diary will give the doctor some insight into your pain and may play a critical role in the management of your disease.

What Will Happen When You First Visit a Doctor for Your Arthritis Pain?

The doctor will usually do the following:
Take your medical history and ask questions such as: How long have you been experiencing pain? How intense is the pain? How often does it occur? What causes it to get worse? What causes it to get better?
Review the medications you are using.

Conduct a physical examination to determine causes of the pain and how this pain is affecting your ability to function.

Take blood and/or urine samples and request necessary laboratory work.

Ask you to get x rays taken or undergo other imaging procedures such as a CAT scan (computerized axial tomography) or MRI (magnetic resonance imaging) to see how much joint damage has been done. Once the doctor has done these things and reviewed the results of any tests or procedures, he or she will discuss the findings with you and design a comprehensive management approach for the pain caused by your osteoarthritis or rheumatoid arthritis.

Who Can Treat Arthritis Pain?

A number of different specialists may be involved in the care of an arthritis patient—often a team approach is used. The team may include doctors who treat people with arthritis (rheumatologists), surgeons (orthopedists), and physical and occupational therapists. Their goal is to treat all aspects of arthritis pain and help you learn to manage your pain. The physician, other health care professionals, and you, the patient, all play an active role in the management of arthritis pain.

How Is Arthritis Pain Treated?

There is no single treatment that applies to all people with arthritis, but rather the doctor will develop a management plan designed to minimize your specific pain and improve the function of your joints. A number of treatments can provide short-term pain relief.

Short-Term Relief

Medications—Because people with osteoarthritis have very little inflammation, pain relievers such as acetaminophen may be effective. Patients with rheumatoid arthritis generally have pain caused by inflammation and often benefit from aspirin or other nonsteroidal anti-inflammatory drugs (NSAIDs) such as ibuprofen.

Heat and cold—The decision to use either heat or cold for arthritis pain depends on the type of arthritis and should be discussed with your doctor or physical therapist. Moist heat, such as a warm bath or shower, or dry heat, such as a heating pad, placed on the painful area of the joint for about 15 minutes may relieve the pain. An ice pack (or a bag of frozen vegetables) wrapped in a towel and placed on the sore area for about 15 minutes may help to reduce swelling and stop the pain. If you have poor circulation, do not use cold packs.

Joint Protection—Using a splint or a brace to allow joints to rest and protect them from injury can be helpful. Your physician or physical therapist can make recommendations.

Transcutaneous electrical nerve stimulation (TENS)—A small TENS device that directs mild electric pulses to nerve endings that lie beneath the skin in the painful area may relieve some arthritis pain. TENS seems to work by blocking pain messages to the brain and by modifying pain perception.

Massage—In this pain-relief approach, a massage therapist will lightly stroke and/or knead the painful muscle. This may increase blood flow and bring warmth to a stressed area. However, arthritis-stressed joints are very sensitive so the therapist must be very familiar with the problems of the disease.

Osteoarthritis and rheumatoid arthritis are chronic diseases that may last a lifetime. Learning how to manage your pain over the long term is an important factor in controlling the disease and maintaining a good quality of life. Following are some sources of long-term pain relief.

Long-Term Relief

Medications

Biological response modifiers—These new drugs used for the treatment of rheumatoid arthritis reduce inflammation in the joints by blocking the reaction of a substance called tumor necrosis factor, an immune system protein involved in immune response system. These drugs include Enbrel and Remicade.

Nonsteroidal anti-inflammatory drugs (NSAIDs)—These are a class of drugs including aspirin and ibuprofen that are used to reduce pain and inflammation and may be used for both short-term and long-term relief in people with osteoarthritis and rheumatoid arthritis. NSAIDs also include COX-2 inhibitors that block and enzyme known to cause an inflammatory response.

Disease-modifying anti-rheumatic drugs (DMARDs)—These are drugs used to treat people with rheumatoid arthritis who have not responded to NSAIDs. Some of these include the new drug Arava and methotrexate, hydroxychloroquine, penicillamine, and gold injections. These drugs are thought to influence and correct abnormalities of the immune system responsible for a disease like rheumatoid arthritis. Treatment with these medications requires careful monitoring by the physician to avoid side effects.

Corticosteroids—These are hormones that are very effective in treating arthritis but cause many side effects. Corticosteroids can be taken by mouth or given by injection. Prednisone is the corticosteroid most often given by mouth to reduce the inflammation of rheumatoid arthritis. In both rheumatoid arthritis and osteoarthritis, the doctor also may inject a corticosteroid into the affected joint to stop pain. Because frequent injections may cause damage to the cartilage, they should only be done once or twice a year.

Other Products—Hyaluronic acid products like Hyalgan and Synvisc mimic a naturally occurring body substance that lubricates the knee joint and permits flexible joint movement without pain. A blood filtering device called the

Prosorba Column is used in some health care facilities for filtering out harmful antibodies in people with severe rheumatoid arthritis.

Weight reduction—Excess pounds put extra stress on weight-bearing joints such as the knees or hips. Studies have shown that overweight women who lost an average of 11 pounds substantially reduced the development of osteoarthritis in their knees. In addition, if osteoarthritis has already affected one knee, weight reduction will reduce the chance of it occurring in the other knee.

Exercise—Swimming, walking, low-impact aerobic exercise, and range-of-motion exercises may reduce joint pain and stiffness. In addition, stretching exercises are helpful. A physical therapist can help plan an exercise program that will give you the most benefit.

Surgery—In select patients with arthritis, surgery may be necessary. The surgeon may perform an operation to remove the synovium (synovectomy), realign the joint (osteotomy), or in advanced cases replace the damaged joint with an artificial one (arthroplasty). Total joint replacement has provided not only dramatic relief from pain but also improvement in motion for many people with arthritis.

What Alternative Therapies May Relieve Arthritis Pain?

Many people seek other ways of treating their disease, such as special diets or supplements. Although these methods may not be harmful in and of themselves, no research to date shows that they help. Some people have tried acupuncture, in which thin needles are inserted at specific points in the body. Others have tried glucosamine and chondroitin sulfate, two natural substances found in and around cartilage cells, for osteoarthritis of the knee.

Some alternative or complementary approaches may help you to cope or reduce some of the stress of living with a chronic illness. If the doctor feels the approach has value and will not harm you, it can be incorporated into your treatment plan. However, it is important not to neglect your regular health care or treatment of serious symptoms.

How Can You Cope With Arthritis Pain?

The long-term goal of pain management is to help you cope with a chronic, often disabling disease. You may be caught in a cycle of pain, depression, and stress. To break out of this cycle, you need to be an active participant with the doctor and other health care professionals in managing your pain. This may include physical therapy, cognitive-behavioral therapy, occupational therapy, biofeedback, relaxation techniques (for example, deep breathing and meditation), and family counseling therapy.

Things You Can Do To Manage Arthritis Pain
Eat a healthy diet
Get 8 to 10 hours of sleep at night.
Keep a daily diary of pain and mood changes to share with your physician.
Choose a caring physician.
Join a support group
Stay informed about new research on managing arthritis pain.

Dietary Supplements

They are products people use in addition to the foods they eat. They include vitamins, minerals, herbs, and amino acids. They are sometimes called "natural" products.

They may come as pills, tablets, capsules, liquids, or powders.
By law, companies that make these products cannot claim they prevent, treat, or cure disease. For example, a product cannot claim that it can "cure cancer" or "treat arthritis."

Can dietary supplements be taken instead of eating certain foods? No

Supplements should not be taken to replace eating a variety of foods. It is important to eat a healthy diet that includes a variety of foods. Dietary supplements are taken to improve the diets of some people. While you need a certain amount of nutrients, too much of some nutrients can cause problems. **Should I check with my doctor before using a supplement? Yes**

If you have health problems and take these products, you may be placing yourself at risk. Persons who are pregnant, nursing a baby, or a have medical problems, such as, diabetes, or high blood pressure, should talk to their doctor first.

Is it safe to take dietary supplements with other medications?
You should talk to your doctor, pharmacist or nurse first. Taking a number of different dietary supplements or using these products together with medication (prescription or over-the-counter) can sometimes have bad effects, even death. Some of these products may also be very bad to take before surgery.

Does the FDA control dietary supplements? No
The FDA does not approve dietary supplements before they are sold.

Companies are in charge of making sure their products are safe before they sell them.

FDA can only judge how safe or effective a supplement is *after* it is for sale.

Then FDA must show that the product is unsafe before it can limit the product's use.

978-0-595-39685-6
0-595-39685-2

www.ingramcontent.com/pod-product-compliance
Lightning Source LLC
Chambersburg PA
CBHW021544290526
45785CB00004BA/1510